Continuing Professional Development in Primary Care

making it happen

Gill Wakley, Ruth Chambers and Steve Field

**Foreword by
Mike Pringle**

*Chairman of Council
RCGP*

Staffordshire
UNIVERSITY

nhs alliance

Radcliffe Medical Press Ltd
18 Marcham Road, Abingdon, Oxon OX14 1AA

British Library Cataloguing in Publication Data

A catalogue record for this book is available from the British Library.

ISBN 1 85775 452 2

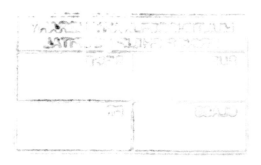

Typeset by Advance Typesetting Ltd, Oxfordshire
Printed and bound by TJ International Ltd, Padstow, Cornwall

Contents

Foreword

This excellent, clear book is the guide we all need. It helps the general practitioner to plan their continuing professional development, to do it most effectively and to record it for clinical governance and revalidation. This book is an essential resource that will be part of the library of every progressive practice.

The most dramatic culture shift facing GPs is the move from continuing medical education (CME) to continuing professional development (CPD). The phrases sound reassuringly similar. The acronyms look interchangeable. However, the reality is that they represent two different paradigms for lifelong learning.

CME is encapsulated in the phrase 'bums on seats'. Although it can be productive, much of it consists of the passive exposure to information that is not directly relevant to the clinical work of the GP audience. The outcome that is measured is not learning or improved care, but the hours of attendance.

It has to be admitted that this was an advance on the previous regimen in which expenses in taking part in education were reimbursed, but there was no incentive equivalent to the Postgraduate Education Allowance (PGEA) to take part. But CME does not encourage personal learning and development.

We all change our clinical practice – in some respects dramatically over short periods of time. When the drivers for change are examined, formal education is relatively modest in its effect. Consider a discussion with a colleague about retinal screening for patients with diabetes followed by an editorial in a journal on the subject – and then reflect on the case of a woman whose vision has been seriously compromised by delayed recognition of diabetic retinopathy. These are the sequences – the triangulations – that most often lead to changes in clinical behaviour.

The advent of CPD recognises this reality and seeks to support and develop it as a legitimate way to develop ourselves and our patient care. It is based on the recognition of educational need; the meeting of that need by the best available means (which might still include the traditional lecture); and the outcome is change in practice and patient care.

If this is just a formalisation of what we all already do, then it should be straightforward. The difficult aspects are the recording of these processes and the embedding of them in our daily clinical lives. To achieve this, we all need signposts, guides and support.

Professor Mike Pringle
Chairman of Council
Royal College of General Practitioners
Professor of General Practice
Division of General Practice
Queens Medical Centre, Nottingham
June 2000

Preface

This book will help GPs, nurses, therapists, practice managers and any other staff learn how to design and apply personal development plans as *individuals* and practice personal and professional development plans as *practice teams*.

The material is also available through Radcliffe Online; the book underpins the online programme and provides a more detailed text for those who prefer to work from a book. The associated book – Chambers R and Wakley G (2000) *Making Clinical Governance Work for You*, Radcliffe Medical Press, Oxford – provides a more detailed text about designing and developing a clinical governance programme.

Health professionals are now expected to approach their continuing professional development in a more systematic way, rather than in the ad hoc manner that has been usual. We should be moving towards team-based learning that includes everyone, whether they are a doctor, nurse, therapist, manager or non-clinical worker. Attached nursing and therapy staff, and other independent contractors, such as community pharmacists, dentists and optometrists, should be drawn into practice educational plans as they evolve.

Individual professional development plans should tie in with practice-based personal and professional development plans. These in turn link into those of the PCG or PCT. The plans will underpin the revalidation of clinicians' professional registration or the accreditation of practices and PCG/PCTs in the future.

The quality of the workforce dictates the quality of healthcare they deliver. Identifying and meeting the education and training needs for the current and future roles and responsibilities of the staff is essential for an effective NHS workforce. This requires resources and a culture that promotes a learning environment throughout the health service.

The future is in multidisciplinary learning together as practice teams. Individual practices will contribute to a coherent plan for the population of their PCG/PCT to provide healthcare relevant to local needs. Practice personal and professional development plans will be a vehicle for the clinical governance programme, taking forward the objectives in the practice's or PCG/PCT's business and development plans.

Practice-based educational plans should equip the practice team members to:

- minimise inequalities in the health of different subgroups of the population
- reduce variations in healthcare services
- define standards for multidisciplinary delivery of care and services
- demonstrate achievements
- sustain quality improvements.

The emphasis in this book is on how you can prioritise what you need to learn. Seven examples are given of plans focused on a variety of clinical and organisational topics, with an integral clinical governance programme running through. You might choose your own topic or follow one of these examples. It doesn't matter where you start, you will find that your learning spreads out to involve your whole practice through the 14 themes of clinical governance presented here.

Gill Wakley
Ruth Chambers
Steve Field
June 2000

About the authors

Ruth Chambers has been a GP for 20 years. Her previous experience has encompassed a wide range of research and educational activities, including stress and the health of doctors, and the quality of healthcare.

She is currently the Professor of Primary Care Development at the School of Health at Staffordshire University. She was the Chair of Staffordshire Medical Audit Advisory Group and a GP trainer for many years. Ruth has initiated and run all types of educational initiatives and activities. She and Gill have run workshops to teach GPs, hospital consultants, nurses, therapists and non-clinical staff about clinical governance. She has also worked with general practices of varying sizes and development to facilitate production of their own educational plans, moving from a rapid appraisal of their baselines to action plans that respond to identified needs. These practice-based personal and professional development plans have involved all members of the practice – doctors, nurses, community pharmacists, employed and attached staff, practice managers and non-clinical support staff. The resulting teamworking has put new heart into the practices concerned.

Gill Wakley started in general practice in 1966, but transferred to community medicine shortly afterwards and then into public health. Her desire for increased contact with patients led to a move back into general practice, together with community gynaecology, in 1978. She has been combining the two, in varying amounts, ever since.

Throughout her career she has been heavily involved in learning and teaching. She was in a training general practice, became an instructing doctor and a regional assessor in family planning, and was until recently a senior clinical lecturer with the Centre for Primary Care at Keele University, Staffordshire. Like Ruth, she has run all types of educational initiatives and activities from individual mentoring and instruction to small group work, plenary lectures, distance learning programmes, workshops and courses for a wide range of health professionals and lay people.

Steve Field is Regional Adviser and Director of Postgraduate GP Education for the West Midlands Region. He is vice-chair of the Committee of GP Education Directors and a member of the national steering group that is implementing the Primary Care CPD Guidance. He has been a GP since 1986 and is a GP principal in inner-city Birmingham. He is also an MRCGP examiner and member of the RCGP's examination board.

List of abbreviations

ACE	angiotensin-converting enzyme
CHD	coronary heart disease
CHI	Commission for Health Improvement
CPD	continuing professional development
CPR	cardiopulmonary resuscitation
CPN	community psychiatric nurse
GMC	General Medical Council
HImP	Health Improvement Programme
IT	information technology
NICE	National Institute for Clinical Excellence
NNT	numbers needed to treat
NSF	National Service Framework
PACT	prescribing and cost data
PCG	primary care group
PCT	primary care trust
PDP	personal development plan
PPDP	personal and professional development plan
RCGP	Royal College of General Practitioners
SWOT	strengths, weaknesses, opportunities and threats
VDRL	Venereal Disease Research Laboratory

Introduction

Where are you now – as an individual or as a primary care team?

YOU ARE HERE if as an *individual* you usually attend courses and educational events:

- as they happen to occur
- if they are held at a time and place to suit you
- if they are held in an attractive venue
- because your friends or colleagues are going
- if the title or speaker takes your fancy rather than because you have identified the topic as a real need of yours
- you rarely think out what you expect to learn from attending the meeting
- you rarely put into practice what you have learnt from a course or a meeting
- you rarely reflect on what you have learnt, later on.

YOU ARE HERE if as a *practice* you do not plan how and what you learn together, so that there is:

- little attempt to identify everyone's learning needs
- no cohesive practice-based personal and professional development plan[1]
- no link between the practice business plan (if it exists) and planned professional development for staff
- no coordination of everyone's learning
- little anticipation of everyone's learning needs if circumstances and requirements change
- an unfair balance of study time and resources for some staff compared to others
- no link between staff appraisals (if they are in place) and professional development
- no consistent link between your practice personal and professional development plan and individuals' personal development plans
- no established learning culture in the practice.

So now YOU ARE HERE this programme will help you rectify these shortcomings. It will guide you though the maze to developing your own:

personal development plans

that will feed into a

practice personal and professional development plan

that will feed into the

education and clinical governance programmes for your

PCG or PCT.

CHAPTER ONE

How to do it: identify your service development needs and your associated learning needs

- As an individual.
- As a practice team.
- As a PCG or PCT.

Get organised as an individual

1   Make your overall learning and development plan – consider the study time needed, commitment, both your own and wider NHS perspectives, motivation, prioritisation and support. Consider how your own personal development plan (PDP) contributes to the wider practice-based planned clinical governance programme.

2   Identify your learning and service development needs – balance your learning needs as an individual and those of your working environment (systems and procedures in your practice, the PCG/PCT, the NHS as a whole). If someone conducted a job appraisal with you in the previous 12 months, see how you can build some of the objectives into your current plan.

3   Look at the PCG/PCT's business plan or the local Health Improvement Programme (HImP). What can you do to contribute to meeting their targets and priorities? You are likely to find that there are more resources for learning or developing those areas in your practice later on.

4   Devise a programme to meet your and your practice's prioritised learning and service development needs. Check it out with someone else to get their perspective on how it fits with the practice as a whole.

5   Select the educational material, making it happen in practice. Choose the courses and events that suit the topic rather than because they are the most convenient or the cheapest in town.

6   Appraise your own learning and development.

7   Evaluate your learning; by yourself or with others. Demonstrate that you are fit to practise. Keep records of what you have achieved.

8   Review the fit between you and your practice; demonstrate that your working environment is fit for you to practise from.

9   Identify new areas of learning – evaluate how you are doing now; anticipate your needs when circumstances change or developments occur for you or your working environment.

Get organised as a workplace or practice team

1   Start with the business plan of the PCG/PCT, or their latest annual plan for clinical governance or primary care investment. If your practice does not have a business plan, draw one up. What are the main areas of service development for the forthcoming year or, looking ahead, for the next three years? The plan should include important NHS priorities such as:
   –   those in the local HImP
   –   recent or expected National Service Frameworks (NSFs)
   –   local priorities such as the conditions for which there are higher-than-average death rates in your local population; particular needs of subgroups of your population, e.g. those from ethnic minority communities
   –   current or anticipated changes in your service delivery, such as if you are developing new models of care with integrated nursing teams.

2   Identify service development needs and staff learning needs using some of the range of methods in the following pages. Decide on the main areas of planned development for which you and other staff will need new knowledge and skills. Consider asking others from outside the practice to comment on whether they think you have framed your service development plan and associated learning programme appropriately. You might ask patients, the public (i.e. non-users of your services), others in the PCG/PCT, local tutors, etc. Define:
   –   short-term objectives for the practice-based personal and professional development plan (PPDP) for the next year
   –   medium-term objectives for up to three years.

3   Identify the learning needs that are essential to deliver your PPDP and clinical governance programmes – balance the clinical and non-clinical needs of individuals and their working environment (systems and procedures in the practice, the PCG/PCT, the NHS as a whole). This balance will include:
   –   generic learning that is relevant for everyone, e.g. communication
   –   team building

－   specific skills for the particular roles and responsibilities of all included in the workplace-based plan.
4   Assess the infrastructure required to deliver your education and training plans for the practice and identify from where you will obtain the necessary resources.
5   When making your overall practice-based learning plan, you'll need to consider:
    －   the staff it involves: GPs, employed nurses and non-clinical staff; does it also include your cleaners, community pharmacists, attached staff and patients?
    －   the extent and resource costs of study time needed: actual costs to individuals and the practice, and also opportunity costs
    －   the practice's and practitioners' commitment
    －   the perspectives and needs of your staff, the practice as a whole, the PCG/PCT, the district and the wider NHS perspectives.
    And how to
    －   motivate the staff
    －   prioritise different learning needs between topics and between staff
    －   support staff and GPs
    －   evaluate what has been achieved
    －   assess and include new learning needs as they arise.
6   Devise the programme to meet the practice's prioritised learning needs; try to give each member of staff a definite role and responsibility to contribute to the overall practice-based plan. The programme should be written out as a timetabled action plan:
    －   a review of the success of previous year's plans and what is still outstanding
    －   how current learning needs will be identified
    －   who needs what and when
    －   how needs will be met
    －   how team members will learn
    －   in-house teaching and learning
    －   reading
    －   meetings or courses outside the practice
    －   applying what has been learned by putting it into practice
    －   practice teamwork
    －   away-day(s)
    －   how and by whom the learning will be evaluated and achievements monitored
    －   how and by whom new learning needs will be identified and included
    －   how any learning is to be disseminated.
7   Make it happen in practice – implement the practice personal and professional development action plan.
8   Evaluate the extent and quality of the service developments and associated learning, and the quality of the learning plan.
    －   Step 1: encourage individuals to self-appraise and evaluate their learning and contribute those reports to the overall evaluation.

- Step 2: evaluate the balance of the learning against the original objectives that were based on the practice business plan and service priorities.
    - Step 3: use comments from patients and external individuals or bodies to evaluate the achievements and direction of the overall plan.
    - Step 4: evaluate the practice-based learning plan itself – was it too ambitious, were there sufficient resources, were all the relevant staff covered, did all the GPs and staff join in?
    - Step 5: how will you change or extend next year's plan?
9   Demonstrate that your working environment is fit for the GPs and practice staff to practise in, with a clear record of what you have achieved: for example, improvements to the quality of patient care, staff wellbeing, effective systems, staff development.
10 Conclude what has still to be addressed and relay to drafting of the next practice PPDP.
11 Disseminate the achievements resulting from your PPDP.

Get organised as a PCG or PCT[1]

1   Review the personal development needs of your board members – to fulfil their roles and responsibilities in the PCG/PCT. These might relate to:
    - management skills to enable them to be effective
    - new knowledge and skills
    - their awareness of national and local policies
    - attitudes to various subgroups of the population or different disciplines and organisations.
    You can see how the various priorities of the individual, the practice and PCG/PCT overlap by referring to Figure 1.1 on page 6.
2   Consider how you will marry the education and training resources and activities in your PCG/PCT with the health needs of the local population:
    - undertake a health needs assessment; seek the advice of those in public health and local government, and the general public in this
    - produce a coherent plan that embraces the general medical practice teams, community-based employees of NHS trusts, other independent contractors, non-health organisations and the general population
    - map out workforce numbers as a whole and per practice; consider whether you have the right balance or if changes should be made.
3   Assess support needs for the practitioners and practices in your constituency: plan how to allocate your resources fairly to various disciplines, clinicians and managers, self-employed and employed or attached staff. Include how you will provide support for your facilitators and tutors in your plan. Seek additional resources.
4   Encourage and enable practices to formulate and execute PPDPs that are centred around priority areas and include as many health professionals, managers and support staff as possible.

5   Devise ways to inform and engage practices about the priorities for the district and their populations, for example:
     –   practical support such as supplying information about morbidity and mortality rates
     –   enhancing information technology (IT) capability and capacity to achieve reliable and accurate data
     –   feeding down national documents and directives to inform their everyday work.

6   Draw up an education and training plan for the PCG or PCT based on the principles outlined in the previous sections. Allocate lines of responsibility, from leadership to delivery. Ensure that it is integral to all other developmental work such as:
     –   clinical governance
     –   monitoring performance
     –   prescribing matters
     –   revalidation and accreditation of practices (such as for training status)
     –   plans for changes to service delivery, the service and financial framework, the business and investment plan.

7   Evaluate the investment in your education and training plan at regular intervals; review and realign the priorities. Challenge historical patterns of education and its delivery – modernise your approach.

8   Develop a close working relationship with your local Non-Medical Education and Training Consortium and Director of Postgraduate General Practice Education to encourage their help and resources in supporting continuing professional development (CPD) in the PCG/PCT.[1]

9   Forge links with local NHS trusts, the health authority, social services and other family health service providers such as optometrists, dentists and pharmacists to break down boundaries between professions for sharing CPD.[1]

10   Encourage community-based NHS trust employees to share their PDPs with the practices with whom they are working so that their individual plans become part of the PPDP.[1]

Stage 1: Make your overall learning plan

Your PDP might form the major part of a future revalidation programme or demonstrate your fitness to practise or manage for you as a GP, nurse, therapist, receptionist or manager. Your plan should:

•   identify your weaknesses in knowledge, skills or attitudes
•   specify topics for learning as a result of changes: in your role, responsibilities, the organisation
•   link into the learning needs of others in your workplace or team of colleagues
•   tie in with the service development priorities of your practice, the PCG/PCT, your district or the NHS as a whole

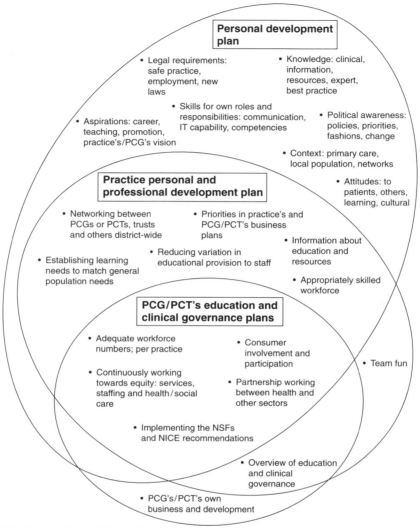

Note: The topics given as priority areas for development are examples and not intended to constitute comprehensive lists.

Figure 1.1 Link your PDP to the PPDP and the educational and clinical governance programmes of the PGC/PCT.

- describe how you identified your learning needs
- prioritise and set your learning needs and associated goals
- justify your selection of learning goals
- describe how you will achieve your goals and over what time period
- describe how you will evaluate learning outcomes.

You will need to set aside enough time to shape and justify your learning plan. The more time you invest in making your plan and the programme of learning, the more likely it is that you will focus your learning effectively. Then you'll spend the precious time that you have, learning about topics that are relevant for your job and for your needs or your practice's needs.

Your PDP

The main task is to capture what you have learned in some way that suits you, so that you can look back at what you have done and:

- reflect on it at a later date, to learn more, make changes as a result, identify further needs
- demonstrate to others that you are fit to practise or work: through what you have done, what you have learnt and what changes you have made as a result; the standards of work you have achieved and are maintaining; how you monitor your performance at work
- use it to show how your personal learning fits in with the practice business and PPDPs.

Organise all the evidence of your learning into a portfolio of some sort

It is up to you how you keep this record of your learning. Examples are:

- *a learning journal* in which you draw up and describe your plan, record how you determined your needs and prioritised them, report why you attended particular educational meetings or courses and what you got out of them, and the continuing cycle of review, making changes and evaluating them
- *an A4 file* with lots of plastic sleeves in which you build up a systematic record of your educational activities in line with your plan
- *a box*: chuck in everything to do with your learning plan as you do it and sort it out into a sensible order every few months with a really good review once a year.

Stage 2: Use a range of methods to identify your learning needs

Where are you now? What are your roles and responsibilities? What do you need to know? What new knowledge, skills and attitudes do you need?

Your learning needs will encompass the context in which you work as well as your knowledge and skills in relation to any particular role or responsibility of your current post. The extent of learning you need to undertake will depend on your level of responsibility for a particular function or task – whether you are personally responsible, you delegate or you contribute.[2] Your learning needs will be different if you practise or work in an inner-city compared with a rural location, or if your practice population has various subgroups, such as the homeless or a preponderance of the elderly, with special needs. Your learning needs should take into account your aspirations for the future too – personal or career development for you, or improvements in the way you deliver care in your practice.

Use several methods to identify your learning needs. No one method will give you reliable information about the gaps in your knowledge, skills or attitudes. It is particularly difficult to determine what it is you 'don't know you don't know' by yourself; yet it is vital that you identify and rectify those gaps. Other people may be able to tell you what you need to learn quite readily. Colleagues from different disciplines could usefully comment on any shortfalls in how your work interfaces with theirs. Patients or people who don't use your services could tell you whether the way you operate or provide services is off-putting. There may be data about your performance or that of your practice that could point out those gaps in your knowledge or skills of which you were previously unaware.

You'll need to use different methods for identifying your learning needs according to your own circumstances, the focus of your learning and which of the 14 themes of professional and service development that make up clinical governance are relevant. Pick out the ones that seem suitable for you and your work situation.

Try to use several different methods for each of the topics that you focus on, so that you get a rounded picture of your needs. In that way you can build up a picture of the gaps you perceive you need to address and those for which there is objective evidence of your learning needs.

Use a range of methods to identify your service development and learning needs

Determine what it is that you 'don't know you don't know' by:

- asking patients, users and non-users of your service
- comparing your performance against best practice
- comparing your performance against objectives in business plans or national directives
- asking colleagues from different disciplines about shortfalls in how your work interfaces with theirs.

Use any or a mix of all of these methods

Use several different methods of identifying service development and learning needs for each area of practice or theme of clinical governance that you focus on, so that you get a rounded picture.

1 Appraise yourself – review how you and your colleagues work

Write down any specific needs that you think you or colleagues have. These will be a mix of skills, knowledge and personal attributes; or new processes for your workplace.[2]

Your, the practice's, the PCG/PCT's aspirations for:
- new models of service delivery
- new roles or responsibilities in the organisation
- the organisation's vision for change.

Your attitudes to:
- other disciplines
- patients
- lifelong learning
- culture
- change.

Context of work:
- networking in health and non-health settings
- team relationships
- different subgroups of the population
- historical service provision
- the organisation's priorities.

Your knowledge:
- clinical
- about your local population
- of best practice
- range of services available locally
- about your organisation
- local experts or other provision
- systems and procedures in your organisation
- inequalities of health or healthcare of your patient population.

Legal requirements:
- health and safety at work
- new legislation
- employment procedures, e.g. equal opportunities
- safe practices, e.g. personal safety.

Awareness of health policies:
- new health policies
- national priorities
- local priorities, e.g. HImP
- fashions, e.g. in clinical practice or how education is delivered.

Skills:
- teamworking and communication
- effective working practices
- your basic competence
- health needs assessment
- practice management
- communication between trusts and PCG/PCTs
- organisational development of your team
- IT and computer capability
- your specialist areas
- planning
- personal management.

2 Ask other people what they think of you: gain feedback from colleagues

Feedback from colleagues or mentors can help you to see what it is that you do not know that you don't know. (Read that again slowly!)

A young practitioners' group met to draw up guidelines about the management of common conditions. They were amazed to discover that at the end of one term they had finished only one subject, such was the variation of opinion they had discovered from researching best practice and talking among themselves.

Workshops, individual mentoring, small groups or just talking with colleagues about how you do your job all help you to assess your needs.

Unless you have some method of recording what you need to learn (or think) about, you will easily forget it in the busy life that you lead. Identifying and using problems that arise naturally in the course of your work help to make it relevant.

Notebooks, a diary or more formal files (paper or computer) help to organise your learning and that of your team. Keep your notebook by you and jot down gaps in your knowledge as events occur.

---

3 Audit methods

Set standards for your performance, find out how you are doing, search to find out best practice, make the changes and then re-audit the care given to patients in the future with the same problem.

- **Case note analysis**. This provides insight into current practice. It can be a retrospective review of a random selection of notes, or a prospective survey of consecutive patients with the same condition as they present.
- **Peer review**. Compare an area of practice with other individual professionals or managers; or compare practice teams as a whole. An independent body might compare all practices in one area, e.g. within a PCG or PCT. This needs to be well-organised so that like is compared with like. Feedback is usually given so that it protects participants' identities. Only the individual person or practice knows their own identity, the rest being anonymised. In a well-established group where there is mutual trust and an open learning culture, peer review does not need to be anonymised and everyone can learn together about making improvements in practice.

When practice A saw that their referral rates for patients with neurological problems were the highest in the 'league table' of local practices, they undertook a retrospective review of the case notes of the last 20 cases referred. Most of the referrals were for advice about the management of migraine. One GP undertook to find out more about best practice and as a result suggested to his partners other steps in patient management that the GPs could take before referring a patient with migraine to a consultant. The GP partners found that the new protocol worked well and most patients with migraine could be managed without referral.

- **Criteria-based audit**. This compares clinical practice with specific standards, guidelines or protocols. Re-audit of changes should demonstrate improvements in the quality of patient care.

You can measure how well your care of diabetic patients is managed by comparing the proportion of patients meeting your criteria for good diabetic care over intervals of time. Consult with all those involved – the patients and carers, chiropodists, nurses, doctors, reception staff, pharmacists, etc. – to improve what you do, put it into action and then re-audit.

- **External audit**. Audit facilitators, prescribing advisers, primary care development managers, etc., can all supply information about indicators of performance which may be useful in carrying out an audit. However, the practice team has to be involved and use the information in an audit capacity. Practice visits from external bodies such as those linked to accreditation for Fellowship by Assessment by the Royal College of General Practitioners (RCGP) or their Quality Practice Assessment programme, or inspection as a GP training practice expose the practice and individual practitioners to external audit.
- **Direct observation**. Record what is observed for later action.
- **Surveys**. Patient satisfaction surveys may seem cheap and easy but their short-comings may outweigh their usefulness. Having set standards you might carry out a survey as a general indicator of care or for detecting a problem rather than as an accurate measure of performance.
- **Tracer criteria**. Assessing the quality of care of a tracer condition may be used to represent the quality of care of other similar conditions or more complex problems. Tracer criteria should be easily defined and measured.

Audit the care of incontinence of your elderly residents in a nursing home as an indicator of the general quality of care of residents of that home.

- **Significant event audit**. Think of a critical incident where a patient or you experienced an adverse event. This might be an unexpected death, an unplanned pregnancy, an avoidable side effect from prescribed medication, a violent attack on a member of staff, or an angry outburst in public by you or a work colleague. You should take the case to a multidisciplinary meeting to reflect and analyse what were the triggers, causes and consequences of the event and if there is anything individuals or the practice as a whole might do to avoid a similar event happening in future.

You *could* undertake a significant event audit as a single practitioner. It is likely to be more effective as a practice team. There will be more opportunity for everyone to be committed to instituting changes in procedures if they have shared the analysis and planned the solution together around real-life examples of patient care. Reviewing individual

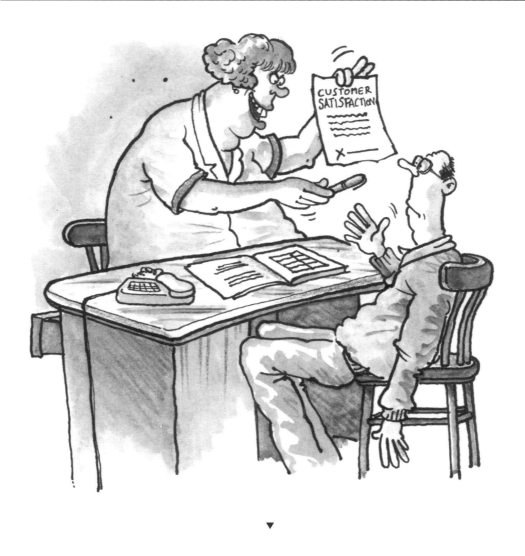

▼

cases in this way will be a test of the learning culture that you have managed to create in the practice. The team does not sit in judgement on any of its members involved in the case. Everyone can learn from any mistakes or omissions that have been made.

STEPS OF A SIGNIFICANT EVENT AUDIT
- Step 1: Describe a critical incident – who was involved, what time of day, what task/activity, the context and any other relevant information.
- Step 2: Recount the effects of the event on the participants and the professionals involved.

- Step 3: Deduce the reasons for the critical event or situation arising, through discussion with other colleagues, review of case notes or other records. Hold discussions to learn from each others' experiences, in supportive manner at dedicated team meetings without interruptions.
- Step 4: Decide how you or others might have behaved differently or approached the issue in another way. Describe your options for how the procedures at work might be changed to reduce or eliminate the triggers or causes from recurring.
- Step 5: Agree any changes that are needed, how they will be implemented, who will be responsible for what and when. You may need to conduct a conventional audit first to assess the extent of a problem to put the significant event in context. Invest time and effort in events that are likely to reoccur or that have a significant impact if they do recur.
- Step 6: Re-audit at a later date to see whether changes to procedures are having the desired effects. Give feedback to the practice team. Acknowledge good care. Specific failures of care (not necessarily ones about which complaints are made, but ones you have identified) can be used to identify a weakness in your personal or team's knowledge, skills or attitudes.

When Mrs S was admitted to hospital in the early hours of the morning with severe congestive cardiac failure the team decided to look at why her heart failure was not picked up when the district nurse was visiting her daily for dressings, so that they could avoid this situation happening in the future. At a meeting of all those involved and from telephone calls to those who could not attend, they found that although her heart condition had been diagnosed, Mrs S had not been reordering the diuretics on her repeat prescription. The doctor had assumed that the district nurse would tell him if Mrs S needed to be seen again. The district nurse thought that the doctor would visit regularly anyway. Neither the prescription clerk nor the pharmacist thought that it was their job to draw anyone's attention to Mrs S's failure to reorder the diuretics. The home carer agreed with Mrs S that she was on too many tablets already and did not understand what the diuretics were for.

An information sheet summarising the illnesses and the care needed was devised and automatically updated by the information put into the computer. A printout was given to patients receiving shared care. They could show this to anyone involved. Audit of a selected number of shared care patients was arranged for 12 months later.

FURTHER READING ON AUDIT

Irvine D and Irvine S (eds) (1997) *Making Sense of Audit* (2e). Radcliffe Medical Press, Oxford. (Out of print.)

Smith R (ed) (1992) *Audit in Action*. BMJ Publishing Group, London.

4 *Monitor your or your practice's clinical decisions*

- Use prescribing and cost data (PACT).

> You want to replace one type of dressing with another. Use PACT data to compare the number of prescriptions for each dressing over several quarters.

- Review the extent to which you adhere to pre-agreed clinical protocols, guidelines and care pathways. Does being unable to justify deviations from the agreed procedures reveal any learning needs?
- Use computer searches.

> You want to ensure that all patients with asthma regularly using a reliever inhaler are also using a preventer inhaler. Compare the results of a computerised search for all those using one type of treatment with another, for all those using both kinds of inhalers. Put your plan into action and monitor with repeat searches at quarterly intervals.

5 *Monitoring the process of obtaining healthcare, i.e. access, availability, satisfaction*

- Access and availability.

> You could look at waiting times to see a health professional by using:
>
> - computerised appointment lists or paper and pen to record the time of arrival, the time of the appointment, the time seen
> - next available appointments which can easily be monitored by computer, or more painfully by manual searches of the appointment books.
>
> Compare the results at intervals.

- Patient satisfaction. You might wish to assess patients' satisfaction with your practice, the PCG/PCT's way of working, or the services available in a locality or a district. Undertaking patient satisfaction surveys was quite a popular pastime for the NHS in the early 1990s when medical audit was being developed. Questions were usually relatively superficial and did not delve into complex areas. A general enquiry may elicit relatively high satisfaction rates; whereas a more specific enquiry might uncover particular elements of dissatisfaction, which will be more useful if you are trying to identify learning needs.

If you undertake a patient satisfaction survey, consider using a tried and tested questionnaire instead of risking producing your own version with ambiguities and flaws.[3,4]

Measure patient satisfaction[5] with consultations, time taken to answer the phone, the quality of information they receive, etc., over time. Use questionnaires or external interviewers. But do beware of the 'halo' effect of patients wishing to please their health professionals by giving less than honest replies.

Other sources of feedback from patients might indicate your learning needs as an individual or as a practice – suggestion boxes or a complete record of all suggestions and complaints from patients, however trivial, looking for patterns in the comments received.

- Referrals to other agencies and hospitals.

You might audit and re-audit time taken from the date the patient is seen to:

- the referral being sent (do you need more secretarial time?)
- the date the patient is seen by the other agency (could the patient be seen elsewhere quicker or do you need to liaise with other agencies over referrals?)
- the date the patient's need has been met by investigation, diagnosis, treatment, provision of aid or support, etc. (can you influence how quickly these are completed?).

You can audit whether referrals are appropriate by the use of proformas or templates.

- Patient complaint. There will be learning to be had from every complaint – even if you are 'squeaky clean' and do not deserve the complaint, there must be something to learn about communication between you and the complainant.

6 Monitoring systems and procedures

Regular problems need action and reviews.

Four staff members were off sick with back trouble at some time in one year. A review of the working conditions showed that two were seated incorrectly at keyboards and new supportive chairs were purchased. One regularly lifted down boxes of dressings from a high shelf and the storage arrangements were changed. The other had injured her back lifting a patient from the floor after the patient had fallen. A back education class was arranged for all the staff as a preventive measure.

Regular team meetings can flag up such problems at an early stage.

> The fire officer found several fire doors propped open. A memo was circulated about this. The manager found no change at an inspection a month afterwards. An investigation showed that staff needed two hands free to pass through the doors. The manager arranged for the doors to be fitted with automatic closures and kick panels at the base instead of handles.

If a problem is not solved the first time, then look at it another way. You may need to seek more information before planning action.

> The valve on the oxygen cylinder was inoperable during a re-accreditation exercise for nurses and doctors on resuscitation. No one had been given the responsibility for checking it, so it had not been checked.

Monitoring systems need to be in place for all equipment. Make sure that there is good data recording of the purchase, arrangements for servicing, and responsibility for maintenance and checking (with deputy arrangements in case of absence or sickness).

Staff health records need to be checked as well and robust systems put into place. Be especially careful when employing locum or temporary staff or with initial employment. Remember to have a routine for checking continued immunity to infection at the recommended intervals. Have you thought of having an occupational health service for your practice or PCG/PCT?

> An antenatal patient developed a rash. The reception clerk for the clinic was a young woman filling in for the regular one while she was on leave. She was found in tears at the end of the clinic – her nephew was thought to have rubella, and she thought she might have given it to the patient. She had not had a check for her rubella immunity before employment because of its transient nature. Fortunately, tests showed that both the patient and the clerk were immune to rubella.

Remember: it's worth recording what you do. Someone, somewhere may want or need to know!

7 Informal conversations – in the corridor, over coffee

It is often said that people learn most on courses when chatting with colleagues at the coffee and meal breaks. This is when you realise that other people are doing things differently from you – and if they seem to be doing it better and achieving more, you can challenge yourself to decide if this matter could be one of your blind spots. Note your thoughts down before you forget them.

Online discussion groups may provide another source of informal exchanges with colleagues.

8 Strengths, weaknesses, opportunities and threats (SWOT) analysis

You can undertake a SWOT analysis of your own performance or that of your practice team or practice organisation, working it out on your own, or with a workmate or mentor, or with a group of colleagues. Brainstorm the strengths, weaknesses, opportunities and threats of the situation.

Strengths and weaknesses of individual practitioners might include: knowledge, experience, expertise, decision making, communication skills, inter-professional relationships, political skills, timekeeping, organisational skills, teaching skills, research skills. Strengths and weaknesses of the practice organisation might relate to most of these aspects too as well as resources – staff, skills, structural.

Opportunities might relate to unexploited potential strengths, expected changes, options for career development pathways, hobbies and interests that might usefully be expanded.

Threats will include factors and circumstances that prevent you from achieving your aims for personal, professional and practice development.

Prioritise important factors. Draw up goals and a timed action plan.

9 Compare your performance with externally set standards

A traditional way of showing that you are competent is to take (and pass) an examination. This is a good way of testing recalled knowledge, but not much good for measuring anything else. A summative examination (i.e. done at the end of a course of study) gives a measure of your learning up to that date.

Passing an examination such as a Certificate of Health Promotion, shows that you know what you should be doing – at least you did on the day you passed!

Doing examination papers where you can look up the answers helps you to learn where to find relevant information. If you remember, or record, this, it helps you to look up other information.

Good Medical Practice for General Practitioners[6] sets out standards of 'excellent' and 'unacceptable' performance. This approach and most of the criteria and standards can be generalised to all health professionals whatever their disciplines. The document expects an excellent GP to meet the excellent criteria all or nearly all of the time; a good GP to meet the excellent GP criteria most of the time; and a poor GP to be consistently or frequently providing care in the unacceptable GP criteria.

You could compare your performance against the criteria listed in this document for:

- clinical practice
- record keeping
- access and availability
- emergency treatments
- out-of-hours care
- keeping up to date
- providing information to patients and colleagues
- professional–patient relationships
- avoiding discrimination and prejudice
- teamwork
- referring patients
- professional ethics
- best practice in research
- effective use of resources
- conflicts of interest
- handling mistakes or complaints.

There are many other assessment programmes with externally set criteria and standards. Standards may be relative, that is referenced to norms, or absolute, that is referenced to criteria.

You might undertake an objective test of your knowledge and skills; for example a computer-based test in the form of multiple choice questions and patient management problems.

10 Observation of your work environment and role

This could be informal and opportunistic, or more systematic, working through a structured check list. One method of self-assessment might be to audio-tape yourself at work dealing with patients (after obtaining patients' informed consent), then listen to the tape afterwards to appraise your communication and consultation skills – on your own or with a friend or colleague.

Look at the equipment in your practice. Do you know how to operate it properly?

Watch yourself undertake practical procedures – do you know what is best practice[7]; are you systematically adopting best practice? Do you make errors or are there unexpected sequelae such as infections – could you learn to improve?

Analyse all the various roles and responsibilities of your current posts. Are you capable of fulfilling these?

Do you know what other colleagues do? How their roles and responsibilities interface with yours? Ask others what they think of your performance. You could ask someone to observe you at work and feedback their opinions in a constructive discussion; then you could repay the favour by reviewing them at work.

You might combine one of the methods of identifying your learning needs already described, such as an audit or SWOT analysis, and apply it to 'observing your work environment or role', describing your relationship with other members of the multi-disciplinary team for example.

11 Reading and reflecting

Try to read articles in respected journals regularly. Actively reflect[8] on what the key messages mean for you in your situation. Note down topics about which you know little, which are relevant to your work.

12 Look at your practice population's health needs and see what you may need to learn as an individual or practice team to address those needs more effectively

Create a detailed profile of your practice population. Ask your PCG/PCT or the local public health department for information about your practice population and comparative information about the general population living in the district – morbidity and mortality statistics, referral patterns, age/sex mix, ethnicity, population trends.

Include information about the wider determinants of health, such as housing, numbers in and types of employment, geographical location, the environment, crime and safety, educational attainment and socioeconomic data. Make a note of any particular health problems, such as higher-than-average teenage pregnancy rates or drug misuse. Focus on the current state of health inequalities within your practice population or between your practice population and the district as a whole.

Consider what you need to learn to reduce inequalities in the NHS care and services that your practice population receives to enable you to plan for anticipated changes in your population, for instance if a series of new nursing homes will mean that you should update your knowledge/skills in elderly care.

You as an individual or a practice team might learn more about the causes of morbidity and mortality of your population so that you can institute a more effective preventative approach. Focus on areas where you can make changes in peoples' behaviour or health status (e.g. smoking cessation) rather than topics that are beyond your direct control (e.g. introducing fluoridation of the water supply).

13 Review the business or development plan of your practice or PCG/PCT and other official strategic documents or directives

Do you know the contents of the key official and informal strategic documents that are relevant to your work? If so, are you aware of the implications and what you need to know or be able to do to make your contribution to achieving the targets set out in these strategies? Note down any gaps to discuss with other colleagues to determine how important it is that you and your practice team take tasks on and whether you have any associated learning needs.

14 *Job appraisal*

Good employment practice includes regular job appraisal, for instance annually. This gives you an opportunity to review how well you are doing in your own view and that of the person who is appraising you. The two of you can agree your learning needs and how they will be met in the context of your current job or agreed changes to your roles and responsibilities.

If you are a senior manager or GP employer you might undertake peer appraisal with another senior colleague whom you trust and whose opinion you respect.

15 *Educational appraisal*

You might find a buddy or work colleague, or a clinical tutor or clinical supervisor with whom you can have a formal discussion about your performance, job situation and learning needs. You might make a learning contract as a result with a timed plan of action.

16 *Review practice protocols and guidelines*

Are you familiar with all the protocols or guidelines that are used by someone, somewhere in the practice? You might determine yours and other practice team members' learning needs by piling all the protocols or guidelines that exist in your practice in a big heap and rationalising them so that you have a common set across the practice. There are bound to be associated learning needs with agreeing a common approach, to enable everyone to be aware of their roles and responsibilities for the various pathways in their everyday work so that they adhere to the protocols or guidelines, or can justify any deviation.

Stage 3: Where do you want to be and how do you get there?

In Stage 2 you found out where you are at present. Now you have to decide where you want to be next.

Think of it as being like a journey to another airport. You know that you are at a major airport. You can go in almost any direction and as far as you like. You may need to change planes, or even the type of transport, but you will only reach the desired destination if you have a plan. If you travel without an aim you will probably end up in the wrong place or even back where you started. There may not be a convenient flight to take you where you want to go or you may not be able to afford the time or the cost of travel. You may need to look for support from others – your work colleagues, the practice team, outside organisations or your personal environment – to achieve your target destination.

Look back at the list of aspirations in Stage 2. Each of the comments you have written for yourself or the practice is a target destination. Try filling in a chart like those below for yourself and the practice team.

From an individual's perspective		
Aspiration	*Destination example*	*Route (see Stage 4 on priority setting)*
Career: from practice nurse to	Nurse practitioner	Professional degree course with support from the practice team and financial support from the health authority or PCG/PCT
Professional development	Certificate in Elderly Care	Work in your own spare time, or in practice time with the encouragement of the practice team or PCG/PCT
Transferable skills	An MA in counselling or an MBA	As above
Personal development	A self-defence course or assertiveness training	As above
Teaching expertise	Become a GP or nurse tutor	A part-time post outside the practice negotiated with the practice team, training on courses and in post
Promotion	Receptionist to deputy practice manager	Professional qualifications at college, time off negotiated with the practice team or in your time
New role or responsibility	Receptionist to audit clerk	Training in practice time, computer skills and IT. Consider if practice team or the PCG/PCT require skills

From the practice's perspective		
Aspiration	*Destination example*	*Route (see Stage 4 on priority setting)*
Organisation's vision for change	Become the provider of XXX services for the PCG/PCT	Training and expertise in XXX, links with secondary care, bid for equipment, support services, accommodation, practice team find time to do it
	Patients to be able to access the practice nurse for advice more easily	Time set aside for telephone consultations, training and computer assistance software program
	Complete audit cycles regularly	Incorporate audit into regular work, train more people, invest in IT to do it easily and automatically, set up regular review meetings and time for all staff to attend relevant areas of audit

continued

	From the practice's perspective	
Aspiration	*Destination example*	*Route (see Stage 4 on priority setting)*
Organisation's vision for change (*continued*)	Set up and run regular multidisciplinary meetings	Someone to organise it, protected time for the staff to attend, IT support and access
	Improve implementation of evidence-based medicine and nursing	Training, education, research involvement, clinical meetings, audit and review procedures; practice or PCG/PCT-based with protected time for activity
	Improve the management of complaints	Training for the complaints manager (practice manager?); systematic review of complaints procedures; comparison with others in the PCG/PCT
	Monitor standards of practice nursing	Training in review, clinical supervision and systematic audit procedures; rectify substandard practice at individual and team levels; training and education
	Develop occupational health scheme for the staff	PCG/PCT to set aside funds for development and employment of suitable personnel
	Improvement of access to clinical records	Standardisation of entry, data, training for IT, new equipment, compare standards across PCG/PCT

Many of the activities of clinical governance are being carried out already. They (just) need coordinating and implementing. Changing performance and improving quality can be difficult, initial enthusiasm for a project to improve quality soon becomes stuck in the daily chores of work. Audit and feedback have been shown to be good ways of changing behaviour. Computer-generated reminders are helpful to keep us all doing it correctly. Have a look at the Cochrane Review on Effective Practice and Organisation of Care[9] and other ways of changing behaviour.[10]

Some people do not want to participate in clinical governance activities, particularly audit. Barriers to participation include:

• fears that clinical governance or audit will be used to shame and blame people
• fears that your own knowledge, skills or performance will be found to be insufficient
• concerns about confidentiality
• concerns that all this activity will not result in any worthwhile change
• worries about taking time away from the real business of medicine (looking after patients).

The best way to convince people that these fears and concerns are groundless is to show them how it all works in practice.

Even then, some will be reluctant or – being human beings – even lazy or pigheaded!

The NHS now has a regulatory body with the power to descend on any NHS establishment – yes, even *yours* – to look at its performance. The Commission for Health Improvement (CHI) will make judgements about the performance of PCGs or PCTs and other NHS trusts.

Now have a go at completing your own chart to inform your own PDP.

Aspiration	Destination	Route (see Stage 4 on priority setting)
Your own perspective		

Aspiration	Destination	Route (see Stage 4 on priority setting)
Career		
Professional development		
Transferable skills		
Personal development		
Teaching expertise		
Promotion		
New role or responsibility		
Other:		
Other:		
Other:		

The practice's perspective		
Aspiration	*Destination*	*Route (see Stage 4 on priority setting)*
Organisation's vision for change		

Stage 4: Setting priorities for what and how you learn

Everyone will have been able to make a wish list after carrying out the previous three stages. The wishes are unlikely to coincide with the needs of the individual, team or organisation. Where they overlap move them to the top of the list!

Pam, the practice secretary, wishes to go on a computer course to learn about spreadsheets and improve her skills. The practice has just bought a new computer dictation package. The practice manager foresees that Pam's secretarial duties of typing letters will diminish. With extra training Pam could take over many of the audit tasks from one of the partners with her new computer skills. Her wishes and the needs of the practice coincide.

Some of the topics on your lists of aspirations will be not be appropriate for the present circumstances, some will be too costly and others too time-consuming. Go through the lists again, selecting those topics that have clear aims and objectives and are achievable within your time and money constraints.

The lists should be more manageable by now, but you will still have more ideas than can possibly be implemented. So you will have to rank them in order of priority.[2]

Imagine that your primary care team or PCG/PCT, or you as an individual, run a picture gallery. You have been sent a large number of pictures and exhibits. You want the critics to acclaim the pictures on display. You may want to sell them or have many red dots of approval put on them. You need to convince others of your wisdom, common sense and business acumen. You would not want everyone who has sent in a picture to decide on whose picture should be hung, so you set up a 'Hanging Committee'.

Who should be on the Hanging Committee to decide which of the topics on your lists of aspirations should be prioritised? It has to be representative and not autocratic or idiosyncratic. In most practices, the practice manager and one or more of the GPs might prioritise the main topics for the PPDP.

But you could choose people to represent the different facets of practice; you might include someone who likes reading and browsing the web to look at research and development, learning and teaching culture, reliable and accurate data, and implementation of evidence-based practice and policy. An intuitive, caring type might want to take on meaningful patient involvement, confidentiality and health promotion. The practice manager is an obvious source of expertise on managing resources and services, risk management and core requirements. That only leaves the overall coordination to the chairman of the committee! Phew – whittled it down to four people.

They would of course, collect information from all the team, the patients, users and carers and feed back the decisions and progress. They must also take into account the

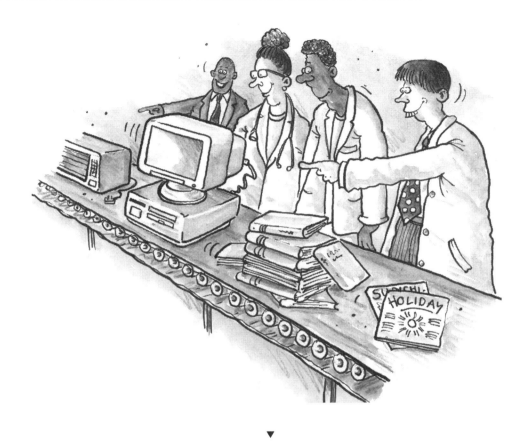

▼

Prioritise your needs as a team.

external influences such as the NSFs, governmental priorities, the district priorities in the HImP, National Institute of Clinical Excellence (NICE), etc.

When ranking topics in order of priority consider:

- whether the project aims and objectives are clearly defined
- it is important:
  - for the population served (e.g. the size of the problem and/or its severity)
  or
  - for the individual/team skills, knowledge or attitudes
- it is feasible
- it is affordable
- it will make enough difference
- it fits in with other priorities.

Think about modifying this list to include your own factors of what is important.

Problems with setting priorities

- There are no clear criteria such as those above, or criteria are used inconsistently.
- The criteria affect each other and are not independent.
- Complex scoring systems are used or spurious numerical values are allocated to the criteria.
- There are too large a number of options at the outset.
- There is a lack of information about the appropriateness or effectiveness of the intervention.
- Reluctance to take decisions that will be unpopular with a vocal minority.
- Reluctance to cut, reduce or ration any existing provision.
- Manipulation of the results for individual gain.
- Judging the benefits to the organisation as a whole versus those for particular individuals.

Remember the highest priority – the health service is for patients that use it or who will do so in the future.

Incorporate the agreed priorities into your own PDP or your practice-based plan. Set dates for completion of the various stages. How will you set standards and evaluate what you have done? You might want to use a table as in the example below.

Improve the management of scabies by increasing self-management by patients: timetabled action plan

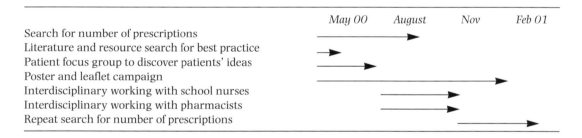

	May 00	August	Nov	Feb 01
Search for number of prescriptions				
Literature and resource search for best practice				
Patient focus group to discover patients' ideas				
Poster and leaflet campaign				
Interdisciplinary working with school nurses				
Interdisciplinary working with pharmacists				
Repeat search for number of prescriptions				

CHAPTER TWO

You have identified your learning needs – now what?

Most of what you will need to know as a health professional or manager who wants to provide high-quality healthcare that is patient-centred and relevant to service needs, follows on here, described as 14 themes of clinical governance.

You might decide to tackle one particular area, such as coronary heart disease, which you perceive as being a priority for the practice. Develop your PDP and PPDP to include most or all of the 14 themes of clinical governance. You might focus on three or four of the seven worked examples presented in the second half of this book and limit the number of themes of clinical governance per topic. Your plans over successive years will fill in the gaps. All your practice learning is likely to flow over into other areas of your work. For instance, if you learn more about 'meaningful involvement of patients and the public', then incorporating the learning into your everyday work should automatically bring you to finding out more about the evidence base for methods of involvement with patients.

How you do it will depend on whether you are using this programme to devise your own PDP, or are working as a practice team on one or more agreed priority areas.

You should complete the template for a PDP on pp. 97–106. It will serve as:

- a personal or practice learning record for you to complete
- an action plan in which to describe how you will meet your learning needs with respect to the topic you prioritise
- a report of what has been achieved and what education and work is still outstanding.

It will probably be easier to copy and complete a template for each main topic as an 'interim' plan, and then finally bring each section of work together into one overarching educational plan for your practice each year.

These record charts have been drawn up in such a way that you can complete them from your own individual perspective and/or that of you and your colleagues and/or your practice. GPs, nurses, therapists and practice managers who have tried out these charts have found that they are easy to use and that they encouraged them to adopt a more structured approach to learning together.

If you are working on your own you will need to be firm with yourself about keeping to the times set out in your action plans and making changes in your everyday practice as a result. It would help you to find a tutor or colleague with whom you can discuss your plan and your progress – to encourage you to keep on track and make sure that you are keeping a balanced perspective on your learning.

Use the same tools to evaluate your progress as you used to identify your learning needs – refer back to the variety of methods described in Stage 2 earlier in the book.

The relationship between clinical governance and professional and service development

Clinical governance underpins professional and service development. Clinical governance 'is doing anything and everything required to maximise quality'.[11] It is about finding ways to 'implement care that works in an environment in which clinical effectiveness can flourish by establishing a facilitatory culture'.[12]

The emphasis is on education and training programmes being relevant to service needs, whether at organisational or individual levels. 'Continuing professional development (CPD) programmes need to meet both the learning needs of individual health professionals and to inspire public confidence in their skills. But importantly they also need to meet the wider service development needs of the NHS'.[13] Not just what you *want* to do, but what you *need* to do.[1]

Lifelong learning and CPD are integral to the concept of clinical governance, and that includes everyone in a practice working towards agreed learning goals that are relevant to service development.

We have identified the following 14 themes as core components of professional and service development, which, taken together, form a comprehensive approach to providing high-quality healthcare services. If you interweave these into your individual and practice personal and professional development plans you will have addressed the requirements for clinical governance at the same time.

They are:

1   Learning culture: in the practice, the PCG/PCT and the NHS at large.
2   Research and development culture: throughout the NHS.
3   Reliable data: in the practice, the PCG/PCT, the NHS as a seamless whole.
4   Well-managed resources and services, as individuals, as a practice, as a PCG/PCT, across the NHS and in conjunction with social care and local authorities.
5   Coherent team: well-integrated teams within a practice, across a practice, in the PCG/PCT.
6   Meaningful involvement of patients and the public: in a practice, the PCG/PCT, the NHS – including users, carers and the general population.

7 Health gain: activities to improve the health of patients in a practice, between practices, in the PCG/PCT, and different geographical areas of the NHS.

8 Confidentiality: of information in consultations, in medical notes, between practitioners.

9 Evidence-based practice and policy: applying it in practice, in the PCG/PCT, in the district, across the NHS.

10 Accountability and performance: for standards, performance of individuals, the practice, PCG/PCT, health authority and the NHS – to the public and those in authority.

11 Core requirements: good fit with skill-mix and whether individuals are competent to do their jobs, communication, workforce numbers, morale at practice level, across the PCG/PCT.

12 Health promotion: for patients, the public – opportunistic and in general, targeting those with most needs.

13 Audit and evaluation: for instance of changes, of individuals' and practices' performance, of PCG/PCT achievements, of district services.

14 Risk management: proactive review, follow-up, risk management, risk reduction.

The aims of the government's programme of modernisation of the health services are to:[13]

1 tackle the causes of ill health
2 make services convenient, quick and easy to use
3 ensure the consistency of services regardless of where you live
4 try and provide joined-up services that are not constrained by artificial barriers between services, such as health and social services
5 invest in improving the workforce and infrastructure.[11]

through:[14]

• clear national standards set by the NSFs and NICE
• local delivery of quality services
• monitoring of services through the CHI
• consultation with patients and the public.

Clinical governance is relevant to all five aims and integral to the delivery of high-quality services in consultation with patients and the public at large. At the heart of clinical governance, and the ultimate aim of any PDP, is minimising inequalities in:

• healthcare: variations in access, service provision or standards of care and discrimination on the grounds of age, gender, ethnicity, sexuality, disability, etc.
• people's health: influenced by risky lifestyles and social determinants of health, such as poor housing or education, low income, transport.

Education and training of the practice team are key planks in any action plan to tackle variations in the delivery of healthcare. The following examples of the components of clinical governance illustrate the wide perspective necessary if the practice team are to reduce inequalities in their daily work.

Health promotion

- *Current inequality*: worried well take up health promotion services disproportionately.
- *What we do now*: opportunistic health promotion, target specific subgroups of the population with respect to coronary heart disease, etc., district disease management committees.
- *What we could do*: the PPDP could promote an integrated approach via primary and secondary care with health promotion facilitators, education and local government sectors, involving the public and voluntary organisations, and helping team members learn how to motivate people to change their lifestyle behaviour.

Meaningful involvement of patients and the public

- *Current inequality*: those that shout the loudest have most impact with individual health professionals and at an organisational level.
- *What we do now*: patchy public involvement; some practices, PCG/PCTs and health authorities run focus groups or patients' representative groups; lay representation at board level may not be consultative.
- *What we could do*: the PPDP could focus on practice team members appreciating the benefits of systematic consultation and public participation in decision making and learning the skills to undertake such consultation so that it is meaningful.

Managing resources and services, e.g. contraceptive services for teenagers

- *Current inequality*: higher rates of pregnancy in socially deprived groups.
- *What we do now*: receptionist training to enable teenagers to access practices more easily, drop-in clinics in practices, young peoples' family planning clinics.
- *What we could do*: the PPDP might focus on finding out what the young people want and need and how to communicate with young people better.

Evidence-based policy and practice

- *Current inequality*: variations in practice and policy are common between practitioners and between practices.
- *What we do now*: allow personal preferences and impulsive choices to override our knowledge of best practice.
- *What we could do*: the PPDP could concentrate on finding ways to apply best practice in real life; enabling all the team members to reach a minimum standard of knowledge and skills; agreeing the roles and responsibilities for the delivery of care for a particular disease or condition.

Risk management

- *Current inequality*: little differentiation in access arrangements for patients with high and low risks (e.g. suicide, asthma).
- *What we do now*: direct access to nurses in some general practices; walk-in centres in some areas; prescribing by some nurses and not others.
- *What we could do*: the PPDP might help team members learn to be more aware of the needs of minority groups – location and timing of provision, language and patient education difficulties.

CHAPTER THREE

Incorporating the 14 components of clinical governance into your PDP and the PPDP

The following sections are abbreviated versions of the full text. The complete text may be found in Chambers R and Wakley G (2000) *Making Clinical Governance Work for You*. Radcliffe Medical Press, Oxford, and on the website of Radcliffe Online: www.primary careonline.co.uk

We have included key points of the 14 themes of clinical governance for you to integrate through your own PDP and that of your PPDP.

1: Establishing and sustaining a learning culture

'Clinical indicators should be used to learn, not to judge'.[15] That this needs stating shows how fragile the learning culture of the NHS really is. Clinical audit has sometimes been used to expose people's shortcomings rather than facilitate learning from experience. League tables of performance have been used out of context to apportion blame; like is not necessarily being compared with like.

Clinical governance will only achieve sustainable health gains and improvements in the quality of healthcare if there is a positive learning culture in the organisation. NHS staff should be able to admit mistakes and call for more resources. Professionals and managers should be able to work and learn together to achieve the standards set out in the NSFs without apportioning blame for shortfalls in service provision.

Applying clinical governance in practice will require a learning culture that encourages:

- a sustained quality improvement culture

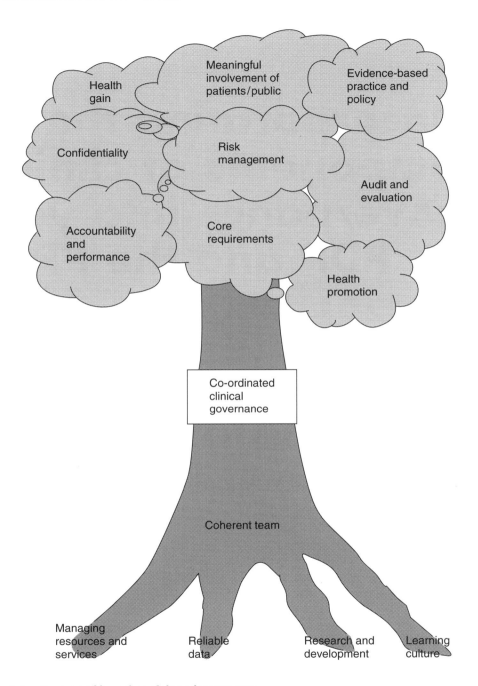

Figure 3.1   Routes and branches of clinical governance.

- evaluation of changes in practice
- reflective practice – learning from experience
- motivated staff
- personal and team development.

Blocks and barriers[16] to establishing a coherent education and training programme across a practice, service, unit, PCG/PCT or trust include:

- isolation of health professionals, even many of those who appear to work in a team
- 'tribalism' as different disciplines protect their traditional roles and responsibilities
- lack of incentives to take up learner-centred, interactive education as opposed to more passive modes of educational delivery
- differing rights to time and funds for continuing education between staff in the same workplace
- lack of communication between health and social care organisations and individuals
- rigid educational budgets for different professions
- practitioners overwhelmed with service work, with little time for continuing education
- dissonance between individuals' perceived educational needs and service relevant needs
- reluctance to develop or accept new models of working and extended roles
- mental ill health: depression, stress, burnout of learner or teacher
- fear of, and resistance to, change.

There is sometimes confusion about the difference between 'education' and 'training'. Education and training can coexist. The two may be differentiated by thinking of:

- education as being about doing things better
- training as being about taking on new tasks.

New learning needs for the NHS workforce are particularly centred around:

- the commissioning and delivery of healthcare that is better informed by local issues and targeted at local health needs, so reducing inequalities
- evidence-based clinical care or health policy, or justifying performance where it diverts from best practice
- working in partnerships with others from various health disciplines, the voluntary sector or local authorities: roles, responsibilities and capabilities of other professionals.

Such areas are complex and require as great an understanding of the context of healthcare as the subject areas themselves. Such learning is achieved by working closely with others, rather than from textbooks or lectures.

The challenge

Does your practice personal and professional development programme:

- have a lead person for education and training for your workforce?

- identify barriers to multidisciplinary learning and working together?
- plan to overcome barriers to shared learning and working as a team?
- ensure that individuals' own educational plans complement and dovetail into the overall business and development plans of the PCG/PCT or other NHS trust?
- balance central and district priorities with individual staff's justified personal and professional development priorities?
- plan to deliver education and training to staff on an equitable basis in ways that are relevant to the topics and staff circumstances?

2: **Managing resources and services**

This involves two overlapping categories:

PEOPLE   and   THINGS.

If you get the people right the organisation will have an excellent basis. You must also make sure that the things you need are in the right place at the right time and working correctly, as well underpinned by well-planned budgets and efficient process management.

Employment law

To manage your staff well, make sure that you provide:

- up-to-date job descriptions
- the terms of employment
- mutual assessment appraisals and individual training and development plans
- training in-house with other staff
- regular meetings with other staff and clear methods of communicating with them at other times
- knowledge of disciplinary and grievance procedures
- personnel records kept securely with access only to authorised people.

Motivating people to do a better job

You cannot praise people unless you know what they are meant to be doing – so be aware of their goals and tasks. You do need to be careful not to become caught up in the details of how they achieve their goals or they will think that you do not trust them to do the job or that you have not made the transition from worker to manager.

The best way to discover what motivates people is to ask them. Some will want more money, others more time, some more flexibility in their work schedule, others more challenging jobs. Observe how each person responds to the rewards you can offer.

Start with the positive and start with the small things. Most of us are not making earth-shattering advances every day, but little achievements and completions. The praise should come:

- immediately after the successful completion of part or all of the task
- from someone who knows what the task involved (not a remote committee)
- from an understanding of what the task involved.

Incentives that work include:

- personal or written congratulations from a respected colleague or immediate superior
- public recognition
- announcement of success at team meetings
- recognising that the last job was well done and asking for an opinion of the next one
- providing specific and frequent feedback (positive first)
- providing information on how the task has affected the performance of the organisation or management of a patient
- encouragement to increase their knowledge and skills to do even better
- making time to listen to ideas, complaints or difficulties
- learning from mistakes and making visible changes.

Clinical governance requires teamworking at all levels of the organisation, with multi-professional consultation, education and training. Managers need to give effective leadership as well as enabling the correct mix of team members. Managers create the culture for change and usually control the resources through which change can occur.

Three-dimensional coordination and management

Think about managing and coordinating in different directions – not only managing and relating to the staff who are responsible to you but in all directions (*see* Figure 3.2).

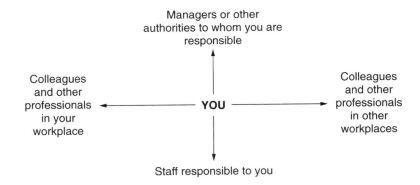

Figure 3.2   Three-dimensional coordination and management.

Think about four levels of change:

- Do we need to do something new?
- Should we do things differently – change a system or process?
- Should we do something different – change the purpose?
- Do we need to stop doing something – does the service or organisation need to exist?

The challenge

Does your practice management link with your practice personal and professional development programme to:

- ensure good management in your practice, with clear lines of accountability?
- promote good communication between management, employers, the grassroots and patients?
- include tried and tested systems for managing change?
- establish a culture where good work is acknowledged and praised?
- offer a proactive approach to sustaining morale and motivation in your workforce?
- check that contracts of employment are equitable between staff in the practice, and between the practice and those who work in the practice but are employed elsewhere?
- provide protected time and resources for appropriate education and training of all your workforce?

3: Establishing and disseminating a research and development culture

A well-established research and development culture in your practice or PCG/PCT that interconnects with secondary care should encourage the wider adoption of evidence-based practice by all practitioners. This in turn should lead to increasingly appropriate patient management and more cost-effective prescribing practices. The NSFs are based on the evidence we have of best practice.

Research and development are essential activities in the understanding of whether or not care is effective and of ways to make best use of resources. But the gap between research findings 'proving' best practice and health professionals and managers applying those findings in their everyday work is considerable and needs to be bridged.

Many clinicians harbour latent desires to do some research in a small way themselves. Any research strategy in the PCG/PCT or practice should harness this enthusiasm for scientific enquiry, while restraining novice researchers from dashing off poorly thought-out studies, which are not completed.

You would be better focusing on 'development' than 'research', unless you have an expert in your practice team or are already part of a research network. Your approach should include:

- understanding how to find out more about the evidence for best practice in investigation, management or treatment in clinical practice or organisational matters
- knowing how to access the findings in published literature and research papers
- establishing an infrastructure with access to the evidence – an up-to-date practice library, staff time to visit the local medical library, links to the Internet and appropriate electronic databases, links to other sources of information about your patient population (public health, mortality and morbidity rates, housing, employment, etc.)
- links to the local university or college as appropriate to your particular areas of interest
- skills training on research methods: for instance, questionnaire surveys or focus groups
- collaborating with others' studies as a way of getting started
- learning about project management, gaining funds, applying for ethical approval
- focusing on topics that are important to your local community: a health issue, a new model of delivery of care
- recording all contacts with patients in a more systematic way to enable you to undertake research on your patient population more readily
- encouraging the integration of evaluation in all aspects of NHS work.

Involvement of consumers in research can have an important influence on the type of research undertaken and the ways in which it is carried out and disseminated. The lay perspective reminds researchers about patients' priorities and values. It keeps the research plan firmly focused on real-life situations.[17]

Critical appraisal

Reading and evaluating a paper is mainly about applying common sense. In general you should consider whether[18,19]:

- the paper is relevant to your own practice
- the research question is clear and well-defined
- any definitions are unambiguous
- the context of the study is described
- the aim(s) and/or objective(s) of the study are clearly stated
- the design and methodology are appropriate for the aim(s) and question posed
- the measuring instruments seem to be reliable; that is, different assessors at different points in time, would make the same observations
- the measuring instruments are valid; that is, the investigator is actually measuring that which s/he intends to measure

- the sampling method is clear
- the outcomes chosen to evaluate any intervention are appropriate
- the results relate to the aim(s) and objective(s) of the study
- the results seem to be robust and justifiable
- the results can be generalised to your own circumstances
- there are any biases in the method of the study or the results, such as non-reporting of drop-outs from the study
- unexpected outcomes are explained
- the conclusions are valid
- you have any other concerns about the study.

The challenge

Does your own PDP or the PPDP:

- include an element of research and/or development as a basic component of your personal or practice development?
- offer staff an opportunity to learn more about undertaking research and seek expert advice?
- provide opportunities for staff to collaborate with experienced researchers?
- enable staff to appreciate the contribution of research and development through skills training in critical appraisal of published literature?

4: Reliable and accurate data

Clinicians, patients and administrators need reliable and accurate data to connect individuals or their healthcare records to other knowledge that is relevant to the care of the patient.

Common problems with data recording in the NHS are that:

- the basic data set of patient identifiers is entered many times over – time and effort are wasted
- the clinical data relating to one episode is not all available in one place, but has to be searched for – sometimes without results
- the opportunity for errors is multiplied each time an entry is made
- it is difficult, if not impossible, to keep accurate and useful records of activity and demand for management and accounting.

Electronic health records can:

- record the information once
- record the information accurately by using templates or on screen prompts

- display the information in a variety of ways, such as a summary, an episode, a chronological account, a stock list, a waiting list or, a priority group for action
- make the information accessible by a variety of people from clinicians, to administrators and policy makers
- make each part of the information subject to different levels of access so that, for example, personal medical information is not available to the accounts clerk
- supplement information not easily available by other means, such as how long people wait when they attend for their appointment
- be consulted remotely across long distances.

A paper record has inherent disadvantages:

- it cannot be in two places at once
- it is difficult to find the information you want in a mass of paper sheets
- it is inefficient – time is wasted looking for the record, looking in the record, copying out information that is in it
- it is bulky and difficult to store efficiently.

Make records easy to use so that you:

- minimise the training needed to use them
- prevent security procedures being circumvented
- record or retrieve information at the correct time
- reduce repetitive routine tasks
- enter or retrieve information in a standardised manner
- facilitate communication between all health staff
- incorporate audit and risk management
- base management and policy decisions on accurate information.

Patient-held records are popular with patients. Smart cards can have different levels of access for different people. For example, a pharmacist could access the medication record but not the results of someone's chest X-ray.

We all grumble about too much paperwork and cannot keep up with the reading that we ought to do. New data gathered in abstract are easily forgotten; what we need is accurate information accessible at the time that the problem presents. Information technology can help:

- search technology can retrieve abstracts of relevant publications
- libraries or user sites can keep you up to date with most of the published data on selected subjects using key words
- best evidence summaries produced by committees of reviewers are published.[20]

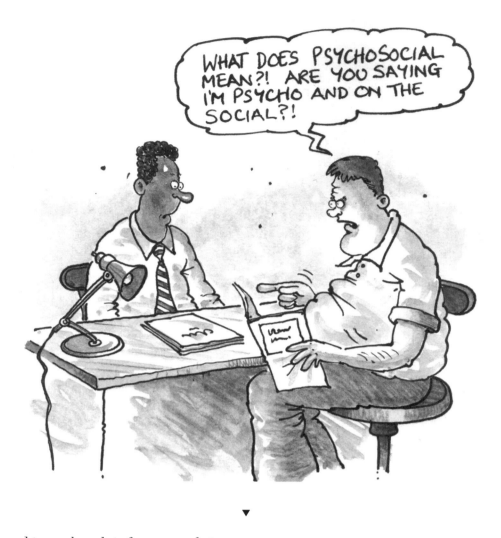

We need to analyse data from records to:

* look at trends and patterns of illness
* devise and use clinical guidelines and decision support systems as part of evidence-based practice
* audit what we are doing
* provide the information on which to base decisions on commissioning and management
* support epidemiology, research and teaching activities.

Standardising entry can be achieved by:

* forms and templates to collect or analyse data
* lists and sets of terms to select; arranging the screen to give prompts to enter data
* structured reports and referrals

- data automatically collected after entry for analysis, audit or departmental reports
- training and feedback to standardise entry requirements.

Patient records are to benefit the patient by providing a record of care that supports the clinician in the present and future care, and provide a medico-legal record to support and demonstrate the competence of the clinician. Increasingly patients receive their care from 'teams' rather than individuals. Without the efficient sharing of information, duplication of effort or even harm may result.

The 'Child's Health Record' for shared recording of encounters with children has been a great success with parents.[21] Parents bring the book to many health professionals and the comments or queries can be seen by all involved in the care of the child, including the parents. They have a record of the child's developmental checks, the written back-up of the advice from the health visitor, and sometimes even reports from the GP. The involvement of the GP has been neglected and many do not understand the purpose or usefulness of the record.

The challenge

Your practice personal and professional development plan should:

- be based on reliable and accurate data: set up systems and training to ensure this – do whatever it takes
- make the most of the potential of your electronic capability for accessing records and monitoring the quality of care
- invest in staff training so that all have a minimum level of competence and capability
- use shared records as a vehicle for multidisciplinary learning.

5: Evidence-based practice and policy

Evidence-based care is the 'conscientious, explicit and judicious use of current best evidence in making decisions about the care of individual patients. The practice of evidence-based medicine means integrating individual clinical expertise with the best available external clinical evidence from systematic research'[22] into everyday work. Clinical effectiveness is successful when linked to local needs and priorities, so long as clinicians, managers, policy makers and patients are all involved in the process.[23]

The evidence base justifying health policy and management decisions in relation to a particular service is just as important as the evidence base for the clinical care component of the service or the education of staff providing that service.

A public opinion poll or demonstrable population needs[24] could provide sufficient evidence to justify providing one service rather than another. These principles are encompassed in the philosophy of clinical governance.

Unless research-based evidence and guidance is incorporated into practice, efforts to improve the quality of care will be wasted. Implementing evidence may require health professionals to change long-held patterns of behaviour.[25]

Measuring clinical effectiveness requires you to work systematically through the following stages.[18]

- Asking the right question – framing it so that it is simple, specific, realistic, important, capable of being answered, owned by those involved, implementable, focused on an area where change is possible.
- Finding the evidence: searching in the published literature, asking experts, etc.[26]
- Weighing up the evidence: as applied to your question in relation to your situation.
- Applying the evidence in practice: involving others, linking practice and policies or strategic plans, getting ownership from work colleagues and managers, overcoming barriers to application.
- Evaluating changes: making refinements to the application of evidence and continuing to monitor performance.
- Applying clinical effectiveness in the wider context of clinical governance.

Information about the effectiveness of a treatment for patients might include[27]:

- the likely effects of a particular intervention
- comparative risks and benefits of one intervention with others
- lay valuations of different outcomes
- clear presentation of probabilities and uncertainties
- discussion of individual applicability
- appropriate inclusions and exclusions – justify range of interventions, options included
- discussion of professional and circumstantial biases.

Patients ought to be well enough informed to be in a position to make rational decisions about their health and healthcare. The better the information patients receive, the better able they are to participate in making decisions about their own clinical management and alternatives.

There is some evidence that well-informed patients who actively share in making decisions about treatment have more favourable health outcomes, for instance in the improved control of the blood sugar levels in the care of diabetics. Giving patients more information has been shown to be associated with greater patient satisfaction too.[28]

The NSFs set out national standards and define service models based on evidence for best practice.

The NSF for Mental Health is aimed at adults up to the age of 65 who have mental health problems. Seven standards have been set for five areas:

1   Health and social services should promote mental health for all.
2   Good primary care and access to services for those with a mental health problem.
3   Effective services for people with severe mental illness.
4   Support and care for carers of those with mental health problems.
5   Action to reduce suicides.

Guidelines at their best, 'assist healthcare professionals ... in more effective practice of the art of medicine'.[29] They promote effective disease management by the 'development and management of treatment programmes for specific conditions in a systematic fashion to optimise the quality and cost-effectiveness of care using the best evidence available'.[28]

The challenge

Does your PPDP:

*   have an evidence base – whether in relation to policy, management or clinical practice?
*   include guidelines that are based on rigorous evidence?
*   measure the effectiveness of development in a way that is meaningful to patient care?
*   address the extent to which the messages you give patients as verbal advice or written instructions are evidence-based?

6: Confidentiality

The principle of confidentiality is basic to the practice of healthcare. Patients attend for healthcare in the belief that the information that they supply, or which is found out about them during investigation or treatment, will be kept secret.

*   Health professionals are responsible to patients with whom they are in a professional relationship for the confidentiality and security of any information obtained.
*   Health professionals must preserve secrecy on all they know. The fundamental principle is that they must not use or disclose any confidential information obtained in the course of their clinical work other than for the clinical care of the patient to whom that information relates.

Exceptions to the above are:

1   if the patient consents
2   if it is in the patient's own interest that information should be disclosed, but it is either impossible or

3   medically undesirable in the patient's own interest, to seek the patient's consent
4   if the law requires (and does not merely permit) the health professional to disclose the information
5   if the health professional has an overriding duty to society to disclose the information
6   if the health professional agrees that disclosure is necessary to safeguard national security
7   if the disclosure is necessary to prevent a serious risk to public health
8   in certain circumstances, for the purposes of medical research.

Health professionals must be able to justify their decision to disclose information without consent. If they are in any doubt, they should consult their professional bodies and colleagues.

Information given to a health professional remains the property of the patient. Generally consent is assumed for the *necessary* sharing of information with other professionals involved with the care of the patient for that episode of care and, where essential, for continuing care. Beyond this, informed consent must be obtained.

Consent is only valid if the patient fully understands the nature and consequences of disclosure. If consent is given, the health worker is responsible for limiting the disclosure to that information for which informed consent has been obtained. The development of modern IT and the increasing amount of multidisciplinary teamwork in patient care make confidentiality difficult to uphold. You should be aware that patients often underestimate the amount of information sharing that occurs.

You may need to give information about a patient to a relative or carer. Normally the consent of the patient should be obtained. Sometimes, the clinical condition of the patient may prevent informed consent being obtained (e.g. unconsciousness or severe illness). There may be exceptional circumstances when a patient should not be given medical information which could be harmful for him or her and the information is given to a relative or carer in the best interests of the patient. It is important to recognise that relatives or carers do *not* have any right to information about the patient.

Reassure young people about their right to confidential medical treatment. Fears about confidentiality are the commonest reason young people give for not attending their GP for contraceptive treatment.[30]

The needs of elderly people or people with disabilities to make their own decisions can often be overlooked. Establish what information they want to be passed on to relatives, carers, social services and others.

Including information about confidentiality in patient leaflets and having notices about confidentiality displayed helps to inform people about the standards you set. Make sure all staff understand the need for confidentiality and explain to patients, each time they ask for information, the rules under which it is given. Many people have not thought about the implications of asking for someone else's results or if they have been seen at the clinic or surgery. You should also ensure that confidentiality is not misused to exclude the patient from decision making.[31]

Occasionally you may feel that your moral duty as a citizen requires you to divulge confidential information. Whenever possible you should seek to persuade the patient to give consent to the disclosure. Seek advice from your professional organisations in circumstances where others are at danger (e.g. risk of harm, rape or sexual abuse), or where a serious crime has been committed. Health professionals should satisfy themselves that sufficient authority has been obtained (e.g. a certificate from the Attorney General or Lord Advocate) and consult professional organisations before disclosing information without a patient's consent.

The Caldicott Committee Report[32] described principles of good practice to safeguard confidentiality when information is being used for non-clinical purposes:

- justify the purpose
- do not use patient-identifiable information unless it is absolutely necessary
- use the minimum necessary patient-identifiable information
- access to patient-identifiable information should be on a strict need-to-know basis
- everyone with access to patient-identifiable information should be aware of his or her responsibilities.

Interpreters should be used wherever possible to avoid the use of friends or relatives. They should be trained in the requirements of confidentiality.

The challenge

Does your PPDP:

- incorporate systems for ensuring that paper and computer security is maintained?
- put into practice systems for monitoring and upgrading security systems?
- systematically check that confidentiality is not being breached if changes are made?

7: Health gain

The two general approaches to improving health are:

1 The 'population approach' focusing on measures to improve health throughout the community.
2 The 'high-risk' approach concentrating on those at highest risk of ill health.

The two approaches are not mutually exclusive and often need to be combined with legislation and community action. Health goals include:

- a good quality of life
- avoiding premature death
- equal opportunities for health.

The Nation's Health: a strategy for the 1990s sets out priority areas and detailed action plans. The authors list eight important general principles for public health strategies:[33]

- partnership between public, professionals and policy makers
- coordination between different organisations
- adequate funding
- long-term planning
- recognising barriers to health promotion
- reducing inequalities in health
- education for health
- research, evaluation and monitoring.

An adequate income for everyone is beyond the remit of health workers, but would have a major impact on public health. It is clear that inequalities of health are closely related to poverty, poor housing and poor education.[34,35] Funding for resources and services is always inadequate compared with what could be done, but good housekeeping means that new demands are subject to a value-for-money test.

Many health improvement plans will not show tangible results for many years. Most avoidable diseases have many causes. Reduction in risks from one factor, e.g. high-cholesterol diets, may not affect cardiovascular disease without tackling other more significant causes, such as smoking. Short-term interventions have been shown to lose their effectiveness rapidly. The HIV campaigns for safe sex were initially successful but later evidence suggested that the effect wore off unless constantly reinforced.[36]

Target setting has some advantages:

- clear monitoring of progress
- a stimulus to set up accurate collection of data
- highlights key aspects of health promotion
- helping health workers to focus on activities related to health policy.

But:

- targets focus on what can be measured rather than on what is important but difficult to quantify
- targets encourage a didactic approach ('big brother knows best'), especially if imposed without sufficient public debate or education about the issues involved
- poor results from poor or inaccurate data, or unrecognised barriers to implementation may be counterproductive
- low morale results from penalising health workers for failing to reach targets which factors outside their control prevent them from reaching.

Even modest gains spread over a large population can have immense health gains for society and individuals. Look at the Cochrane review on the effectiveness of advice for smoking cessation.[37] Individual efforts of advice on smoking cessation targeted at health service users need to be coupled with population-directed health promotion activities. These include governmental measures such as taxation, control of sales, health warnings, control of advertising, funding for health promotion and smoking cessation programmes. The evidence for health gain for smoking cessation is clear. Other lifestyle changes are not so obviously beneficial.

We use screening tests to try to detect illness before it develops. Wilson's criteria[38] help us to decide whether screening is worthwhile (*see* Clarke and Croft,[39] as in the box).

Wilson's criteria for screening: TRAP WILSON

Treatable condition
Resources for screening and treatment available
Activity must be continuous
Audit cycle continued
Protocols needed for a clear policy on when to treat
Worthwhile (cost versus benefit)
Important to individual and community
Latent phase exists for detection before disease develops
Suitable and acceptable test
Outcome improved by detection
Natural history well understood

The challenge

Will your PPDPs:

* result in health gains for many that are sustained?
* have realistic expectations of health gains that can be made from your planned actions?
* be applicable to 'hard-to-reach' groups of people, to improve their health?

8: Coherent teamwork

Teams do produce better patient care than single practitioners operating in a fragmented way.[40] Effective teams make the most of the different contributions of individual clinical disciplines in delivering patient care. The characteristics of effective teams are:

* shared ownership of a common purpose
* clear goals for the contributions each discipline makes
* open communication between team members
* offering opportunities for team members to enhance their skills.

A team approach helps different team members adopt an evidence-based approach to patient care – by having to justify their approach to the rest of the team.[40]

The experiences of teamwork on the Wirral[40]

The team was composed by including a family support worker employed by the voluntary sector into a community psychiatric nurses team. They found that the factors that helped the team to work well were:

- that each member of the team had a separate function
- joint training helped to cement the team; but obstacles from different employer arrangements had to be overcome
- interdisciplinary differences of opinion about patient care were welcomed as a way of increasing debate and generating a wider range of options for care.

The themes[41] emerging to shape the future of healthcare delivery focus on teams with:

- boundaries between primary and secondary care disappearing
- more integrated care
- easier access to primary care
- an increased range of healthcare services provided by primary care practitioners
- an increasingly multidisciplinary primary care workforce
- nurses with extended skills, responsibilities and training
- continuing gatekeeping responsibilities in primary care
- greater integration between health and social services planning and provision.

Clinical governance will be practised at a service level[42] through multidisciplinary teams working across agencies. Teams that encourage participation are more likely to achieve a patient-centred service, to work together as a team and be more efficient.[42]

What predicts the effectiveness of primary healthcare teams?[43]

A study of 68 primary healthcare teams in the UK found that team size, tenure and budget-holding status did not predict team effectiveness. The most effective teams had clear objectives, encouraged participation from its members, emphasised quality and supported innovation.

Good communication is essential for good teamwork.[44] You need:

- regular staff meetings – where managers and staff endeavour to attend
- a failsafe system for passing important messages on
- a way to share news so that everyone is notified of changes as soon as the information is available
- opportunities for quieter members of the team to contribute
- to give and receive feedback on how your role in the team is working out
- everyone to be part of and own the decision making.

Team building starts from the top. Managers and senior clinicians should set good examples that encourage trust and respect from other colleagues. Without this, no organisation will be able to function at its full potential. This takes time, effort and consistency but you'll reap the rewards.

Clinical teams

Integrated nursing teams have existed for years but interdisciplinary teams require more development.[45] In a clinical team where members may have overlapping clinical responsibilities, make clear and unambiguous handover arrangements. Consider:

- who leads a multidisciplinary group
- how you find out who to contact
- how you reconcile different priorities and perspectives
- how to overcome difficulties people have in working together.

Include nurses, doctors, paramedics, pharmacists, therapists and other operational staff and clinical leads in clinical improvement teams. Consider how best to involve the public in your decisions.[3]

The challenge

Does your PPDP:

- involve all members of the team?
- have clear goals and objectives that are owned by all members of the team?
- allot specific roles and responsibilities to team members, and do they know what these are?
- include action to feedback news and results to team members?
- recognise the contributions and achievements of all team members in the clinical governance effort?

9: Audit and evaluation

Audit is 'the method used by health professionals to assess, evaluate and improve the care of patients in a systematic way to enhance their health and quality of life'.[46] The five steps of the audit cycle are to:

1   Describe the criteria and standards you are trying to achieve.
2   Measure your current performance of how well you are providing care or services in an objective way.

3   Compare your performance against criteria and standards.
4   Identify the need for change – to performance, adjustment of criteria or standards, resources, available data.
5   Make any required changes as necessary and re-audit later.

Performance is often broken down into the three aspects of structure, process and outcome for the purposes of audit; this approach was recommended by Donabedian.[47]

Structural audits might concern resources such as equipment, premises, skills, people, etc. Process audits focus on what was done to the patient, for instance clinical protocols and guidelines. Audits of outcomes consider the impact of care or services on the patient and might include patient satisfaction, health gains, effectiveness of care or services.

The direction of clinical audit should be to promote:

- a clear patient focus
- greater multiprofessional working
- an intersectoral approach across primary, secondary and continuing care boundaries
- close links with education and professional development
- the integration of information about clinical effectiveness, cost effectiveness, variations in practice, outcome measurement and critical appraisal skills.[48]

Evaluation

Setting up evaluation of a new service change or model of delivery is complicated by the fact that the outcome may be dependent on many factors other than your own initiative, or it may take many years to see results.

Other ways of incorporating evaluation into your everyday work might be by:

- performance management: to check that the project or service fulfils predetermined criteria of achievement
- external review: undertaken by an independent expert
- internal review: undertaken by members of the project or service providers themselves
- peer review: undertaken by peers in your field.

Undertaking audit

Quality may be subdivided into eight components: equity, access, acceptability and responsiveness, appropriateness, communication, continuity, effectiveness and efficiency.[49] You might use the matrix below as a way of ordering your approach to auditing a particular topic[50] with the eight aspects of quality on the vertical axis and structure, process and outcome on the horizontal axis. In this way you can generate up to 24 aspects of a particular topic. You might then focus on several aspects to look at the quality of patient care or services from various angles.

Matrix for carrying out an audit

For example, if the topic was diabetic care, you might look at the process of communicating results to patients, whether patients from 'hard-to-reach' groups have equal access to your routine diabetic clinic or if the outcome of management is equally effective whether patients are seen in routine GP surgeries compared to a nurse-run chronic disease clinic.

	structure	process	outcome
equity			
access	young people/clinics		
acceptability and responsiveness			
appropriateness			
communication		blood results	
continuity			
effectiveness			HbA1c in GP versus nurse clinics
efficiency			

The challenge

You might design your PDP or your PPDP after detecting problem areas following an audit of:

- the range of provision of services – specialist services in particular settings; choice of doctor/nurse; prevention and treatment
- appropriateness of services provided – extent to which services meet local needs
- accessibility of services – where located, opening times
- information – type, options for non-English speakers
- knowledge – extent to which the public are aware of type and availability of services
- skill-mix – staffing levels
- training of staff – working within competence, sufficient opportunities for CPD
- good employer practices for staff – regular appraisal, regard for health of staff at work, good communication with staff at all levels
- whether underlying reasons for failure to meet standards were identified.

10: Meaningful patient and public involvement

You must be sincere about wanting to involve patients and the public in making decisions about their own care or about local health services for such an exercise to be successful. Real consultation involves a shift of power. Until you are ready for that, any public involvement in decision making will be a token event. If people feel that their opinions matter and their views are valued and incorporated in the decisions that are made they will be more likely to cooperate again in the future.

Involvement may occur at three levels: (i) for individual patients about their own care, (ii) for patients and the public about the range and quality of health services on offer, and (iii) in planning and organising health service developments.

The phrase 'patient and public involvement' is used here to mean individual involvement as a user, patient or carer; or public involvement that includes the processes of consultation and participation.[3]

The NHS Executive[51] believes that:

- services are more likely to be appropriate and effective if based on needs identified together with users (and the public)
- users are seeking more openness and accountability
- patients want more information about their health condition, treatment and care
- involving patients in their own care may improve healthcare outcomes and increase patient satisfaction
- patients need access to reliable and relevant information to be able to assess clinical effectiveness themselves

---

If a patient involvement or public consultation exercise is to be meaningful it has to involve people who represent the section of the population that the exercise is about. You must find ways to seek out the opinions of ordinary people who haven't got time to go to meetings or the inclination to fill in survey forms. People in 'hard-to-reach' groups, such as the homeless or those who speak little or no English, will be most unlikely to come forward and give their views unless you use an intermediary. You will have to set up systems to actively seek out and involve people from minority groups or those with sensory impairments, such as blind and deaf people.

Don't just do a survey or run a focus group because it seems a good idea or there is a requirement to do it, or it will end up being a meaningless exercise. Before you start: define the purpose, be realistic about the magnitude of the planned exercise, select an appropriate method or several methods depending on the target population and your resources, get the commitment of everyone who will be affected by the exercise, frame the method in accordance with your perspective, write the protocol.

You might choose one or more methods of involvement from the alternative methods set out as a flowchart below. The information from two or three methods may be combined to give you a better picture of patients' and the public's views.

If your target population is

Practice population or local community | Patient group, patients, carers
↓ | ↓
Interactive process | Interactive process

Options:
- consensus development conference
- Delphi study
- public meeting
- citizens' jury
- lay representative on board as conduit
- presentations to groups, discussions
- talk with Community Health Council
- public notices
- prize-winning competition
- advertise board meetings well to public

Options:
- lend videos
- sit in on users' group as observer
- run nominal groups
- give presentations to users' groups
- invite comments on draft plan
- involve users in evaluating service
- patient record diaries
- hand-held patients' records

Patients/public receive information

Patients receive information

Options:
- hold discussion on local radio
- hold roadshow
- health information booklet to households
- work through voluntary organisations to hard-to-reach groups

Options:
- particular patient/group give lay perspective
- create library of resources for patients
- lay people act as advocates
- organise coordinated cascade
- advisory notices about changes
- use other's communication system
- start correspondence in local newspaper

Patients/public give information

Patients give you information

Options:
- set up and use standing panel
- one-off opinion poll
- focus groups
- semi-structured interviews
- neighbourhood forums
- rapid appraisal initiative

Options:
- community development project
- focus groups
- nominal groups
- face-to-face interviews
- feedback or evaluation slips

Figure 3.3   Making difficult decisions about treatment, funding or resources.[3]

11: Health promotion

Different approaches to health promotion include:

*   medical and preventative behaviour change
*   educational
*   empowerment of the individual
*   social change.

The health service is mainly concerned with the medical model that aims to reduce morbidity and premature mortality. You need to consider how you can inform patients about health risks and how you can help patients change their behaviour.

Table 3.1 below summarises one model for health education.[53]

Table 3.1:   Model for health education

---

1   **Health persuasion**: interventions by professionals aimed at individuals, e.g. advice to stop smoking or take exercise

2   **Legislative action**: interventions by professionals aimed at communities, e.g. lobbying for legal sex education programme changes in school

3   **Personal counselling**: led by individual need performed by professionals, e.g. professionals helping an individual choose treatments when options are available

4   **Community action**: led by community needs performed by professionals, e.g. professionals helping a group to lobby for a local resource

---

You can target whole populations, e.g. giving advice on the prevention of depression to everyone you see or you can target high-risk groups, e.g. giving advice on the prevention of depression to elderly people with precipitating causes such as bereavement.

The medical approach can be criticised for ignoring the social and environmental aspects of disease. It tends to encourage dependency on medical knowledge and can remove health decisions from individuals. Health professionals need to develop strategies to encourage individual action (empowerment) and reduce attitudes of coercion or blame.

The essential nature of health education is that it is voluntary. If patients attend for advice or treatment for a particular problem, is it right to include opportunistic information gathering in the consultation? Patients may not have given their *full informed consent* to these activities.

Access to health promotion activities is often difficult for those with physical handicaps, visual or hearing impairment, etc. Think about how to provide informational materials other than in traditional leaflet format.

Monitoring of activity may be all that can be achieved, but you should be clear about the differences between monitoring and evaluation.

The value of health checks, regardless of health status, is not clear. There are few screening activities that have benefits clearly based on evidence rather than hope. Those who would benefit most from lifestyle advice are least likely to take up services on offer. Those who need to make the greatest lifestyle changes often have environmental

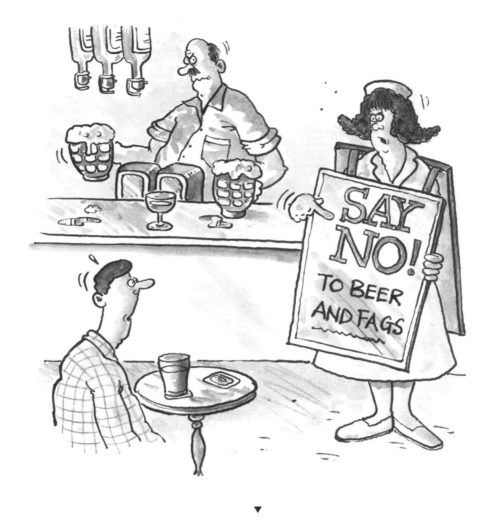

▼

constraints, such as poverty or poor housing, which are mainly susceptible to political or community changes.

Challenges for you about undertaking health promotion

- Are you enabling people to direct their own lives?
- Do you respect people's decisions even if they conflict with your own?
- Do you treat people equally?
- Do you work with people on the basis that those who need your help most come first?
- Are you doing more good than harm?
- Are you telling the truth and keeping promises?
- Will your actions increase the health of the individual?

- Will your actions increase the health of a particular group?
- Will your actions increase the health of society?
- Will your actions have any effect on your own health?

The challenge

Does your PPDP take into account:

- any legal aspects relating to health promotion?
- 'know-how' on risk assessment of health promotion interventions?
- knowing which interventions are the most effective and efficient action?
- being certain of the evidence on which interventions are based?
- the views and wishes of those involved in providing health promotion?
- the views and wishes of those receiving health promotion?
- preliminary work to justify the action plan?

12: Risk management

Your PCG/PCT or other NHS trust is accountable for delivering minimum standards of care through clinical governance. Risk management detects deficiencies, then applies strategies that establish standards and minimise shortfalls in the provision of care and services. Good organisation and efficient practice systems should reduce the chances of mistakes happening or patients not being followed up.

Risks may be prevented, avoided, minimised or managed where they cannot be reduced.

Health and safety in primary care – risk assessment and risk reduction

An employer's duty[54] is to:

- make the workplace safe and without risks to health – of staff or visiting patients
- ensure that articles and substances are moved, stored and used safely
- provide adequate welfare facilities
- inform, instruct, train and supervise staff as necessary for their health and safety
- keep dust, fumes and noise under control
- ensure plant and machinery are safe and that safe systems of work are set and followed
- draw up a health and safety policy statement if there are five or more employees, and make staff aware of the policy and arrangements
- provide adequate first aid facilities.

Innovation – and risk taking

Innovation involves an element of risk taking and uncertainty. The vision of the community trust/primary care model of the future with different types of provision will not be possible if the workforce is not sufficiently flexible and willing to adapt to different ways of working. Retention of staff is very important if the innovation is to succeed for if staff are not supported in change management, a proportion will leave.

The vision for how primary care might develop in the future bears such risks[41] as:

- the potential loss of the 'personal touch' for patients as some primary care is provided via telephone helplines and IT
- loss of continuity of care as a trade-off for offering patients more convenient and faster access to primary care advice and information
- insufficient capacity in primary care to meet the expanded range of services envisaged
- staffing, structures and budgets that are not sufficiently flexible to achieve innovative models of service delivery while retaining uniformly high-quality primary care.

Controlling risk factors

The magnitude of risk is derived from the 'likelihood' and the 'severity' of negative outcomes happening.[55] When people weigh up a risk and make a conscious decision about whether to take that risk they:

- identify the possible options
- identify the consequences or outcomes that might follow from each of those options
- evaluate the desirability of each consequence
- estimate the likelihood of each consequence associated with a specific option
- combine these steps to make a decision – taking into account their own preferences and habitual behaviour.

People usually have a reasonable idea of the *relative risks* of various activities and behaviours, although their estimates of the *magnitude* of risks tend to be biased – small probabilities are often overestimated and large probabilities are often overestimated. But people may underestimate a risk when they apply relative risks to themselves and their own behaviour – for example, many smokers accept the relationship between smoking tobacco and disease, but do not believe that they are personally at risk. People claim that they are less likely than their peers to suffer harm, which makes it less likely that they take precautions. Thus if you wish to modify people's behaviour so that they adopt less risky lifestyles, you should not only provide information about risk but also reinforce your messages by engaging the person in considering the costs and benefits of the behavioural alternatives.[55]

Relative risk is deduced from comparing the effects of being 'highly' exposed to the risk factor as opposed to being 'slightly' or not at all exposed to that factor. There is a proportional change in the risk of a disease for a given change in the level of the risk factor.

Relative risks[56]

These are often used to compare a population group exposed to a suspected risk with a control group. The ratio of the two incidence rates provides the relative risk of the event occurring in one population group compared to another:

$$\text{Relative risk} = \frac{\text{Incidence rate A}}{\text{Incidence rate B.}}$$

A relative risk close to 1.0 suggests no association between exposure and the outcome (such as a disease).

The challenge

Your PPDP should:

- incorporate risk management for every major topic of your programme
- help staff understand the difference between relative and absolute risks of the conditions, lifestyle factors, etc., considered for varying types of patients
- address risks to staff as well as patients, e.g. their personal safety, overload from work, burnout from excessive change
- include how to relay the concept of 'risk' to patients such that the impact of the message changes their subsequent behaviour.

13: Accountability and performance

Clinical governance requires all providers of healthcare to have robust and effective systems for ensuring the quality of their services. These should meet national clinical standards. Standards promoted through the NSFs or in guidance from the NICE should achieve a more uniform quality of care across the country in future.

Local quality monitoring should detect unacceptable variations in performance of practices or practitioners. Those responsible for clinical governance should explore the reasons for substandard performance, offer education and practical support, and require action to rectify shortfalls and improve the quality of healthcare.

Health professionals are accountable to:[57]

- the general public, who are entitled to expect high standards of healthcare
- the profession, to maintain standards of knowledge and skills of the profession as a whole

- the government and employer, who expect high standards of healthcare from the workforce.

Accreditation in healthcare is a system of review using external standards. Standards may be set nationally and checked locally, or set locally and checked by a national body. Accreditation has been directed at the organisation and management of hospitals rather than the clinical competence of doctors and other health professionals. There are moves to incorporate clinical audit and clinical guidelines into accreditation.[58]

Accreditation has five key characteristics:[58]

- review of the performance or capacity to perform (e.g. with respect to a hospital, practice or practitioner)
- external involvement of a statutory or professional body and/or peers
- standards to do with aspects of performance or capacity to be assessed and the values or circumstance that are expected
- measurement of performance or capacity to perform against those standards
- report of results – whether performance is at accepted level with recommendations for action.

Performance

There are six components in the NHS performance assessment framework:[59]

- health improvement
- fair access
- efficiency
- effective delivery of appropriate care
- user/carer experience
- health outcomes.

Clinical governance, professional self-regulation and lifelong learning are the three corner-stones in achieving high-quality healthcare.[60] The CHI will help to maintain standards of care through its monitoring function. A broad range of performance indicators should be developed through the NHS Performance Framework to identify indicators that are appropriate for effective monitoring of whether care is of high quality.

What kind of performance patients want

The aspects of care that are most highly valued by patients are:[61]

- availability and accessibility of care – appointments, reasonable waiting times, good physical access, ready telephone access
- technical competence – health professional's knowledge and skills, effectiveness of professional's treatment

- communication – time to listen and explain, give information and share in decisions
- interpersonal factors such as health professional being humane, caring, supportive and trustworthy
- good organisation of care – continuity, coordination, near location of services.

In considering the priority to be given to a particular treatment or service, the four dimensions of *effectiveness*, *value*, *impact* and *efficiency* should be taken into account as well as the public's preferences and views.[62]

- Effectiveness is the extent to which a treatment or other healthcare intervention achieves a desired effect.
- Value is a judgement made by an appropriate group as to how valuable that effect is in one patient relative to the value of other treatments. Quality-adjusted life years (QALYs) are one way of measuring value.
- Impact is the value of an effect weighted for the degree of effectiveness. A treatment or intervention with a high impact will be highly effective and the effect will be considered very valuable by most people (for example extend life by a reasonable amount, good reduction of pain, etc.).
- Efficiency is the cost of the treatment or intervention for a particular level of impact.

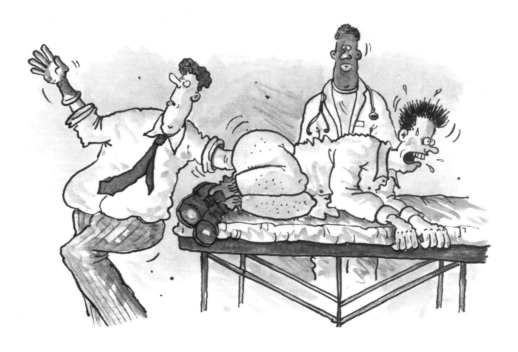

▼

Be aware of the limits of your competence.

The challenge

Your PPDP should allow you:

- to demonstrate the performance of team members and the practice organisation as a whole
- to be sure who is accountable for what, how and when for designing and delivering the programme
- to improve your knowledge, skills and attitudes in responding to patients' views and priorities
- to detect underperformance of staff members.

14: Core requirements

Clinical governance will be a challenge for organisations and staff. It requires a shift in culture, in particular:

- education and training focused on organisational needs and on the needs of the individual
- adequate resources to provide time for the work and for the training
- the identification and development of leaders in every sector
- the development of a 'non-blaming' culture within an organisation.

Well-trained and competent staff

1   Staff need to be:
    - correctly qualified to do the job when appointed
    or
    - correctly trained to an assessed competence before working without supervision.
2   Every staff member should have a PDP supported by the management.
3   Identify the education and training needs (not wants) according to:
    - the requirements of the service
    - identified individual deficiencies in knowledge, skills or attitudes.
4   Education and training should be provided in-house or elsewhere and the time to do this supported.

You should review performance continuously by audit to establish competence and identify attitude problems or gaps in knowledge or skills.

People carry out inappropriate tasks because:

- it has always been done that way
- there is no one else to do it

- no one has thought about the best way to do it
- they enjoy doing that job.

> The development of a practice-based, self-contained community nursing team prompted a reconsideration of how best to make use of the available skill-mix. The nursing auxiliary was trained to offer venepuncture to housebound patients to increase the availability of specialised nursing time.

The NHS Executive supports the vision of new 'nursing role' substitutes for the doctor as doctors' hours are reduced. But if nurses become more and more qualified and specialised, who will do the basic nursing role[63]?

Nurses taking on responsibilities outside their traditional role must ensure that the tasks are:

- in the patient's best interest
- within their personal skill and competence
- carried out after an enhancement of their knowledge or skills
- not compromising their existing duties
- best carried out by them and not by others with different roles or skills
- organised so that they are able to be personally accountable for their actions.

Cost-effectiveness

Cost-effectiveness is not synonymous with 'cheap'. A cost-effective intervention is one which gives a better or equivalent benefit from the intervention in question for lower or equivalent cost, or where the relative improvement in outcome is higher than the relative difference in cost. In other words, being cost-effective means having the best outcomes for the least input. Using the term 'cost-effective' implies that you have considered potential alternatives.

An intervention must first be considered *clinically* effective to warrant investigation into its potential to be *cost*-effective. Evidence-based practice must incorporate clinical judgement. You have to interpret the evidence when it comes to applying it to individual patients, whether it be evidence about clinical effectiveness or cost-effectiveness. A new or alternative treatment or intervention should be compared directly with the next best treatment or intervention.

An economic evaluation is a comparative analysis of two or more alternatives in terms of their costs and consequences. There are four different types: cost-effectiveness, cost minimisation, cost utility and cost-benefit analyses. Cost-effectiveness analysis is used to compare the effectiveness of two interventions with the same treatment objectives. Cost minimisation compares the costs of alternative treatments which have identical health outcomes. Cost utility analysis enables the effects of alternative interventions to be measured against a combination of life expectancy and quality of life; a common outcome measure being QALYs.

Efficiency is sometimes confused with effectiveness. Being efficient means obtaining the most quality from the least expenditure, or the required level of quality for the least expenditure. To measure efficiency you need to make a judgement about the level of quality of the 'purchase' and be able to relate it to 'price'. 'Price' alone does not measure efficiency. Quality is the indicator used in combination with price to assess if something is more efficient. So, cost-effectiveness is a measure of efficiency and suggests that costs have been related to effectiveness.

The challenge

Does your PPDP:

* look at whether the current skill-mix in your team is appropriate?
* explore more cost-effective alternative types of delivery of care?
* include a sufficient focus on staff training for those taking on new roles and responsibilities?

CHAPTER FOUR

Carrying out your action plan: finding appropriate ways to learn

The basis of the learning environment you'll need to create to carry out your plans is about staff learning together as a team. This applies whether the team works in a small unit such as a single-handed general practice, or a much larger team such as in a multi-partner practice where different disciplines may work as subteams within the whole. The education and training plan for the team should address service, and individuals' development; the strategy should focus on ways of implementing the education and development plan and overcoming barriers to its application.

New educational requirements of today's NHS

- making education and training plans that complement those of the unit or practice, PCG/PCT or other NHS trust, district and central priorities
- the implementation of clinical governance: knowledge, positive attitudes, new skills and a learning culture
- adoption of evidence-based practice and policy: where and how to get the information, how to apply the evidence and monitor changes
- needs assessments: how to do them, who to work with, link with commissioning, ways to reduce health inequalities
- working in partnerships with: other disciplines, clinicians and managers, clinicians and patients or the public, non-health organisations
- how best to involve the public and patients in decision making
- understanding and working with new models of delivery of care
- delivering tangible 'health gains' rather than improvements in structures and systems
- encouraging a culture whereby research and development are inextricably linked

---

Learning to work in partnerships

You learn about working in partnerships with others from various health disciplines, the voluntary sector or local authorities by working closely together.

The traditional approach to education in the NHS has been to segregate the professions. This is no longer tenable. Service changes affect everyone and a coordinated approach will be needed at the local level if the health service is to deliver new models of care that are better targeted at the needs of the community.

Preliminary work[64] establishing the education and training needs of GPs and community nurses in the Oxford region found that respondents wanted to learn more about team-working, planning and management, and public health skills. Networking between PCG/PCTs and other NHS trusts allows the sharing of 'ideas, experiences and functions'.

Continuing education and development plans in practice

In a telephone survey of 100 general practices in 1999, 73% of responding practices had continuing education and development plans for practice staff; 27% had assessed staff training needs in the previous 12 months. Education and training needs were not identified by risk management or audit. Neither practice development activities nor district-wide education for GPs were directed at local population health needs or priorities.[65]

People choose to learn in ways that they are used to, or are most convenient rather than the most appropriate for the topic they need to learn about

A recent survey of the education and training needs showed how health professionals and managers opted for the mode of training with which they were most familiar (usually a lecture or validated professional course) or suited their working conditions (for example distance learning for those who found it as difficult to take study leave from their workplace as pharmacists do). Few matched their educational requirements with the mode of delivery that was most appropriate for the topic.[66]

Lectures are only useful for transferring knowledge. If active discussion is an essential part of learning then you would be better joining in small group work and interactive discussion. Most of the new requirements of learning for the NHS require a change of attitudes and deeper understanding of others' views or experiences – difficult concepts to transmit via lectures.

Problem solving and thinking are effective approaches to learning. The seven stages are:[67]

- clarify terms and concepts in the problem
- define the problem – set out what needs to be understood
- analyse the problem – generate possible explanations
- make a systematic inventory of the explanations – link ideas
- formulate learning questions – what you need to be able to understand
- collect information – try to find the answers
- synthesise and test the information – test your answers and discuss the findings.

Learning about such complex subjects as clinical governance or teamworking involves:

- cultural change
- flexibility to adapt to new roles and responsibilities
- negotiation and political awareness.

Education about clinical governance could be by a mix of paper-based activities, electronic newsletters, workshops, lectures, seminars and tutorials. Activities should be as interactive as possible to encourage a deeper understanding of the issues, and the consequences of action or omission. People learn in different ways; a variety of methods of education and training allow people to opt for the methods by which they are more readily engaged and learn best.

Criteria for successful learning[68]

The most successful CPD involves learning which:

- is based on what is already familiar to the learner
- is led by the learner's own identified needs
- is problem-centred
- involves active participation by the learner
- uses the learner's own resources – built on their previous experiences
- includes relevant and timely feedback
- is given when the learner experiences the need to know something
- includes self-assessment.

Lifelong learning combines formal and informal learning as a natural part of everyone's everyday lives. Strong links between theory (the teaching), practice and health policy should ensure that lifelong learning applied to the NHS is relevant to service needs.

CHAPTER FIVE

Multidisciplinary learning: what does it mean in practice?

Potential benefits of multidisciplinary learning include:[68–70]

- opportunities to develop a more appropriate skill mix of healthcare professionals
- the development of new roles
- professionals working together in an atmosphere of openness and trust
- real communication between the team members
- an appreciation of the strengths of the diversity of other staff
- respect for others' professional judgement
- a common set of values and attitudes
- an understanding of each other's roles and responsibilities; and how different professions and staff work best together.

Uniprofessional education still has a place. Some clinical or organisational subjects are so specialised that they only apply to one particular discipline or subspecialty of doctors, nurses or therapists, and peoples' learning needs will be different.

The types of barriers which obstruct multiprofessional learning are:[70]

- a lack of time – often used by doctors as an excuse for not attending in-house training
- the medical model which inhibits 'multiperspective communication'
- organisational structures and processes – making collaborative practice difficult to maintain
- mistaken assumptions about the meaning of multiprofessional learning being about topics that are common to everyone, rather than being about the different professions contributing to a coordinated team.

An example of multidisciplinary learning

A general medical practice closes the surgery once a month to all but emergency cases for organised educational meetings. All staff are encouraged to attend in paid time, so there is a good turn out from the GPs, practice nurses, the practice manager, ancillary staff, district nurses, health visitors and other attached staff, if the topic is appropriate. On the last occasion the team focused on coronary heart disease and handling emergency situations. All staff brushed up on cardiopulmonary resuscitation (CPR), and planned their roles and responsibilities in response to various emergencies. The receptionists learnt about who and how to prioritise with telephone triage, the practice manager learnt more about equipment and procedures, the nurses and doctors learnt about risk management and prevention of acute episodes, and updated their knowledge of best practice.

CHAPTER SIX

Personal development planning

We have prepared two worked examples of PDPs in this chapter:

1   dementia
2   information technology.

These examples are not meant to be comprehensive and you could modify them to match your own ideas and circumstances. Alternatively, if these topics do not emerge as part of your learning needs use them as a guide to writing your own PDP.

The pages of key facts should describe the sort of information and sources of reference that should be useful in justifying that particular topic as a priority issue or as a benchmark by which to compare how you or your practice fares. We cite publications that carry information about the original references, rather than the specific references themselves, for simplicity.

Each example is based on one topic; you might find that this is all you can manage in the course of one year, especially if you widen your programme around the various components of clinical governance that you incorporate into your plan. For instance, considering 'confidentiality' matters in relation to passing on or withholding information about patients with dementia, might lead you to focus on the whole issue of 'confidentiality' in some depth as applicable to other conditions or situations.

The worked examples are followed by a template for you to prepare your own plan. Demonstrate what you have achieved and keep a learning record.

A PDP should contain:[1]

*   a priority topic justified by your previous needs assessment
*   an action plan
*   measure of baseline and follow-up level of knowledge, skills, attitudes, etc. to allow evaluation of learning
*   methods of learning relevant to topic
*   how learning is incorporated into everyday practice and disseminated to others
*   further learning required.

Worked examples

A PDP focusing on a mental health topic: dementia

Who chose topic?

You may have chosen it yourself out of a personal interest in care of the elderly – for example a close family member might have developed Alzheimer's disease, or your practice or PCG/PCT might have encouraged you to learn more about the topic for any of the reasons given below.

Why topic is a priority

(i) A personal/professional priority? You may realise that you are not up to date in developments in the management of dementia when you were unable to justify why you would not prescribe a new drug for dementia when asked to do so by the family of a patient with dementia.

(ii) A practice priority? You may be anticipating a new nursing home being opened in your locality and want to prepare the practice team.

(iii) A district/national priority? There are an increasing number of elderly people in the population of which a considerable proportion will develop dementia.

Who will be included in your personal development plan?

You might involve:

- GPs
- social workers
- practice nurses; district nurses; health visitors
- local psychiatrist
- voluntary organisation representative, e.g. of the local Carers' Association
- practice manager
- receptionists
- community psychiatric nurse
- community pharmacist
- carers of those with dementia
- other agencies who might help, e.g. housing associations, citizens' advice bureau.

You might find out more about each of their roles and responsibilities; or organise a multi-disciplinary learning event; or simply be aware of who is who and where you and patients can contact them in your locality.

What baseline information will you collect and how?

- Numbers of patients with dementia on your practice list. If your practice classifies people's conditions and enters them on the computer then a simple search should yield the numbers. If you do not have a 'disease register' you may need to compile a list by hand with all practice staff contributing names. Map out how many live in residential or nursing homes and how many live in the community.

continued

- Audit extent of proactive and reactive care received by those with dementia. See how many have had their hearing and sight checked in last two years or been reviewed to see if they are incontinent and if so need help or aids.
- Identity of providers of health and social care for those with dementia.
- Any information on morbidity or mortality of those with dementia that your local public health department can supply.
- Any protocol or guide available in the practice or in the district in relation to assessment and management of dementia.
- Any literature for those with dementia or their carers.
- Any survey or monitoring exercise undertaken in the practice in respect of those with dementia.

How will you identify your learning needs?

- Use the checklists and methods for identifying learning needs in the earlier section of this book. For example, you might see how you fare against a protocol of best practice – can you distinguish whether a patient has dementia or just early memory loss?
- You might hold a practice meeting with all those involved in providing care as listed above and agree a more effective model for service delivery. They will have learning needs too, associated with any newly allotted roles and responsibilities.
- Get feedback from the carers of those with dementia by simply asking them what you or the practice as a whole can do better.
- A significant event audit conducted on someone with dementia who is taken to the Accident and Emergency department by exasperated neighbours and dumped there may reveal learning needs for you and the rest of the practice team.

What are the learning needs for the practice and how do they match your needs?
You may find that everyone in the practice realises that managing dementia more effectively is a priority for the practice; or you might find that you're on your own in wanting to learn more and change practice. You will need the commitment of the practice team if you are going to do any more than change your own management and practice.

Any patient or public input to your plan?
You could usefully ask the representative from the local branch of the voluntary Carers' Association or individual carers themselves for their views and suggestions for improvements in helping those with dementia to receive as much practical help as possible. You might do this through talking informally, holding a focus group or organising an open evening with some education and networking as well as gaining their input directly into your plans.

   You or someone else from the practice might sit in on a meeting of a local voluntary organisation or neighbourhood forum where dementia is on the agenda. You should pick up tips for what you need to learn like that.

How you might integrate the 14 components of clinical governance into your PDP focusing on the topic of dementia

Establishing a learning culture: you might hold an open evening for carers of those with dementia to discuss, using a question and answer format, what practical help they need; you might invite a social worker or continence nurse to give a short talk.

Managing resources and services: knowing who else might provide practical and social care to those with dementia or their carers, what they can offer, where to find them and when, e.g. financial advisers in local citizens' advice bureau.

Establishing a research and development culture: you might critically appraise the latest key paper on prescription drugs for dementia.

Reliable and accurate data: know how many people with dementia are registered with your practice and whether they live in the community. Are they on medication that might exacerbate their health problems? Look up the side effects of drugs they are taking.

Evidence-based practice and policy: find out and apply the evidence for selecting appropriate tests to classify someone as having dementia. Can you, for instance, use the 'Mini-Mental' test (see 'key facts' page) in a primary care environment or is it only meant for hospital outpatients?

Confidentiality: know the rules about divulging confidential information about a person (the one with dementia) to another (e.g. their carer or a volunteer in the community) without their express permission and informed consent.

Health gain: learning more about concurrent physical problems that occur in those with dementia (such as urinary infections causing incontinence, undetected deafness) and treating those problems effectively will result in considerable health gains for the patients.

Coherent team: understand everyone's roles and responsibilities in managing dementia effectively as a multidisciplinary team, and the capability of other members of the team of which you might have been previously unaware.

Audit and evaluation: audit the number of people with dementia who are followed up in the practice or undertake a significant event audit. You might audit adherence to a practice protocol for the management of dementia, identifying the gaps in care for which you are responsible and your learning needs to fill them.

Meaningful involvement of patients and the public: learn what methods can be used to engage people with dementia or their carers in a meaningful way, so that they can influence decision making.

Health promotion: target carers for health promotion. Find out what problems they usually develop – it is very stressful and hard work caring for someone with dementia 24 hours a day.

Risk management: learn more about reducing the risks of overprescribing or keeping the patient safe from harm, such as from elder abuse.

Accountability and performance: learn how to construct and present your 'portfolio of evidence' demonstrating that you are looking after people with dementia along the lines laid out in the practice protocol or the good practice that you adopt.

Core requirements: could a different skill-mix in your practice team provide more cost-effective care of those with dementia? You may have to learn more about skill-mix first.

Aims of your PDP after preliminary data-gathering exercise

To provide effective management of those with dementia within currently available resources
[and/or]
to determine a more effective approach to providing care of those with dementia in your practice
[and/or]
to learn more about the clinical management of people with dementia and apply that learning in practice.

Action plan (include objectives, timetabled action, expected outcomes)
Who is involved/setting: you in the general practice setting, plus anyone else in the practice team or associated with it, with whom you might work.

Timetabled action: start date
By xx month: preliminary data gathering completed and staff involved:

*   is there a protocol for managing patients with dementia?
*   numbers of staff; map expertise; list other providers
*   referral patterns and prescribing patterns
*   information about characteristics of practice population, known performance of providing care, local and national priorities.

By xy month: review current performance:

*   extent of knowledge and usage of practice protocol for managing dementia; whether it is it based on best practice and fits with others' management plans (e.g. hospital trust) audit of actual performance via pre-agreed criteria, e.g. assessing newly diagnosed patients
*   compare performance with any or several of the 14 components of clinical governance.

By yy month: identify solutions and associated training needs:

*   learn how to detect people with dementia earlier
*   write or revise the practice protocol on the management of dementia having searched for other evidence-based protocols; input from practice team and psychiatrist
*   clarify your role and responsibilities for caring for people with dementia
*   apply the protocol, identify gaps in care, propose changes to others at practice meeting
*   attend external course or in-house training as appropriate.

By yz month: make changes:

*   feedback information to practice manager to relay to PCG/PCT to justify request for more resources
*   improve access, find ways to prioritise patients with dementia
*   increase referrals to voluntary sector.

Expected outcomes: more effective management of dementia; greater detection of concurrent problems from proactive approach; reduction in overprescribing; increased help from those in voluntary sector.

How does your PDP tie in with your other strategic plans?
(for example the practice's business, or personal and professional development plans, the Primary Care Investment Plan)

It should tie in with the practice's development plan and the PCG/PCT's development plan as far as possible. The PCG/PCT plans should in turn match with the local HImP, social services and other NHS trusts' strategic developments.

What additional resources will you require to execute your plan and from where do you hope to obtain them?
You might ask the practice to sponsor the costs of obtaining literature of best practice. Your entitlement to reimbursement of course fees or time spent on education and training will depend on who you are/your post, and the terms and conditions in your contract. Also on whether the practice perceives that dementia is a priority for the practice team and you are undertaking work on the practice's behalf.

How will you evaluate your PDP?
You should use similar methods to those you used to identify your learning needs as given in Chapter 1, e.g. you might re-audit a topic in which you believe you have made changes and improved your performance.

How will you know when you have achieved your objectives?
You can re-audit the care and services you have focused on 12 months later that relate to the objectives you defined at the outset.

How will you disseminate the learning from your plan to the rest of the practice team and patients? How will you sustain your new-found knowledge or skills?
You might share what you have learnt at the local Carers' Association members' meeting; at a practice educational meeting to the rest of the practice team; or by writing an article for the medical press on effective management of dementia in primary care.

How will you handle new learning requirements as they crop up?
Jot down any thoughts you have about what else you need to learn as you discover it – or you will not be able to remember what it was you were going to look up later on.

Key facts about dementia that you might use to justify the topic as a priority to incorporate in your PDP

- Two out of five GPs use protocols or tests to diagnose dementia.[71]
- Less than half of GPs believe that they have sufficient training to identify and manage dementia.
- The value of prescribing currently available cholinesterase inhibitors for dementia is uncertain. Small observable improvements in behaviour or functional ability may not be clinically relevant; and it is not clear how to assess which patients will benefit.[72]
- An approximate breakdown of the causes of dementia are: Alzheimer's disease (55%), vascular dementia (20%), Lewy body disease (15%), Pick's disease and frontal lobe dementia (5%) and other dementias (5%).[73]
- About 5% of all people aged 65 years and above, living in the community, have a dementia. The rate increases with age such that one in five people aged 80 years and over will develop a dementing illness.[73] Different studies report different prevalence rates mostly explained by using different methodology and criteria for identifying and classifying people.[74]
- Memory loss is the cardinal sign of dementia.
- Features suggestive of Alzheimer's disease include: prominent and progressive memory impairment, conversational problems reflecting word-finding difficulties, disorientation in place, especially if surroundings are unfamiliar and global cognitive impairment.
- Depression and personality disorder can be mistaken for dementia.
- Depression can coexist with dementia.
- Referral guidelines might cover: diagnosis, treatment, management of behavioural disturbance, needs of the carer, long-term placement in residential, nursing or psychiatric care.
- A Mini-Mental State Examination might be used as a brief, standardised cognitive test to assess the patient.[75]
- Reversible dementia is only found in 1% of patients assessed in memory clinics.[76]
- Typical screening tests for people for whom you suspect dementia are: full blood count, ESR, B_{12} and folate assay, VDRL, urea, creatinine and electrolytes, glucose, thyroid function tests, calcium and phosphate, electrocardiogram, mid-stream urine and urinanalysis.[76]
- Enquire about and treat coexisting incontinence.
- Thinking of risk management consider risks to which person suffering from dementia is exposed in their home setting: falls, wandering, fire, hazards, driving, over-sedation from prescribed medication.[76]

Check out whether the topic you choose to learn is a priority and the way in which you plan to learn about it is appropriate

---

Your topic: dementia

How have you identified your learning need(s)?

a	PCG/PCT requirement	X	*e*	Appraisal need	❒
b	Practice business plan	❒	*f*	New to post	❒
c	Legal mandatory requirement	❒	*g*	Individual decision	❒
d	Job requirement	X	*h*	Patient feedback	X
			i	Other	❒

Have you discussed or planned your learning needs with anyone else?
Yes   X   No   ❒   If so, who? *Other GPs*

What are the learning need(s) and/or objective(s) in terms of:
Knowledge: What new information do you hope to gain to help you do this?

To learn more about when to start treatment with newly developed drugs

Skills: What should you be able to do differently as a result of undertaking this learning in your development plan?

Identify people suffering from dementia earlier on in the course of their illness

Behaviour/professional practice: How will this impact on the way you then do things?

I might become the 'expert' in our practice about dementia; and use assessment tests for people whom any of the practice team suspect has dementia

Details and date of desired development activity: *Within three months: attend a day course locally on managing dementia. Within six months: sit in on a dementia assessment clinic with local consultant specialising in elderly care, spend a few hours in local day centre that caters for those with dementia and talk to social carers, more reading*

Details of any previous training and/or experience you have in this area/dates:
Nil, I'm ashamed to say!

Your current performance in this area against the requirements of your job:
Need significant development in this area ❒   Need some development in this area X
Satisfactory in this area   ❒   Do well in this area   ❒

Level of job relevance this area has to your role and responsibilities:

Has no relevance to job	❐	Has some relevance	❐
Relevant to job	❐	Very relevant	X
Essential to job	❐		

Describe how the proposed education/training is relevant to your job:
Integral part of my work caring for elderly people

Additional support in identifying a suitable development activity?
Yes   X   No   ❐

What do you need? *To know when and where relevant courses are being held. Help in learning to search the literature for key papers*

Describe the differences or improvements for you, your practice, PCG/PCT or employing NHS trust as a result of undertaking this activity:
My newly found expertise will be useful to others; I will be raising the standards of care we offer people with dementia in our practice and I will be more aware of what help and support other agencies can offer patients, referring patients as appropriate

Determine the priority of your proposed educational/training activity:
Urgent   ❐   High   X   Medium   ❐   Low   ❐

Describe how the proposed activity will meet your learning needs rather than any other type of course or training on the topic:
The mix of learning from a day's course and personal learning by observing others' everyday practice in different settings should help me to identify what I don't know and meet my learning needs

If you had a free choice would you want to learn this? **Yes**/No
If **no**, why not? (please circle all that apply):
waste of time
already done it
not relevant to my work, career goals
other

If **yes**, what reasons are most important to you (put in rank order):

improve my performance	1
increase my knowledge	3
get promotion	
just interested	
be better than my colleagues	
do a more interesting job	2
be more confident	4
it will help me	

Record of your learning about dementia

You would add the date, length of time spent etc. on each learning activity

	Activity 1: knowledge of best practice in management of dementia	Activity 2: learning skills of identifying and classifying people with dementia	Activity 3: more aware of help and support services from non-NHS agencies	Activity 4
In-house formal learning				
External courses	Day course at local postgraduate centre			
Informal and personal	Sit in with hospital consultant in dementia clinic Reading and reflecting	Discuss criteria used with hospital consultant and staff in dementia clinic; use their assessment scales that are relevant to primary care Reading	Spend time observing in day centre Talk to social care workers Read literature from voluntary sector and social services	
Qualifications and/or experience gained	Experiences of others at course; and other initiatives in the literature	Experience of secondary care procedures	Experience of social care centres	

A PDP focusing on information technology

Who chose it?
It might be your own choice or that of someone in the practice or PCG/PCT team who thinks that you should have additional skills in IT.

Why topic is a priority
(i) A personal or professional priority? You may have chosen IT seeing a need for it yourself or as an inevitable development in your work. You may have agreed as part of your work development, or as a requirement of a change in work duties or responsibilities. You may have volunteered after development in IT was identified as a practice or PCG/PCT need.

(ii) A practice priority? Perhaps the practice has identified that you have not been entering data or that the practice annual report would be easier to prepare if everyone enters data in a consistent way. You may want to introduce a computerised patient call system. The practice may want to use IT for another project or for audit but has insufficient IT skills available, or the practice is preparing to become 'paperless'. Patient need may have increased the number of computerised protocols in use. The practice may have a need for an in-house expert in hardware or software to reduce support bills.

(iii) A district priority? The PCG/PCT may need more data than can be supplied by paper records, or they may need additional expertise. Electronic links with health authorities and hospital trusts are becoming increasingly important. The health authority may have a commitment to have all practices connected to NHSnet within a certain time framework and a Local Implementation Strategy that includes other IT projects.

(iv) A national priority? The government wants to see all practices connected to the NHSnet. It wants you to be able to communicate with secondary care for quicker transmission of patient information and for making appointments at the time the patient is referred. It expects health professionals to be able to take advantage of the Internet opportunities for retrieval of up-to-date information.

Who will be included in your personal development plan?
You might like to find others who want to increase their skills. Working together or as a cascade of learning from each other makes learning more cost-effective and standardisation of data entry is improved (provided you do not pass on faulty habits!). Learning skills and then passing them on makes for more effective learning for you too.

Everyone needs to have the opportunity – reception staff, practice manager, secretaries, *all* the health professionals and anyone who is going to enter anything on your computer system. You might want to offer computer-based health information to patients as well or use patients as a resource. Remember confidentiality and security issues.

You may want to consider IT training as a PCG/PCT activity to ensure consistency, exchange skills and reduce costs. Bringing in outside experts in IT training then becomes more cost-effective and can be tailor-made for the particular needs of the learning group.

continued overleaf

Who will collect the baseline information and how?
You could ask the practice manager or secretary to find out, or the IT lead at the PCG/PCT, or the health authority IT adviser for details of IT training available. If you are already Internet connected you can search for other, more distant, information yourself. You may have a useful health informatics department at a local university or based at a hospital trust. Your computer supplier may provide training – your data entry clerk may know.

You need to know what computer systems are being used in the workplace – the PCG/PCT or health authority may already have collected this information.

Find out from the IT adviser what is in the pipeline for the immediate and long-term future development of IT in your area.

How will you identify your learning needs?
Use the checklists in the earlier sections of the book. Among other methods you might want to do a SWOT analysis.

Strengths and weaknesses: enthusiasm; a logical mind; willingness to go on learning (IT changes rapidly); communication skills and inter-professional relationships to enable interdisciplinary working; organisational, teaching skills, research skills to provide a resource for IT once learned; user-friendly and well-designed software and hardware in the practice, with sufficient spare capacity for quality improvements.

Opportunities: a relative or friend with IT skills; an in-practice expert; a recent IT learner who is enthusiastic to pass on his or her newly acquired knowledge; expertise at home computing on which you can build for professional proficiency; a decision to gain a qualification in IT, finding a local course of interest, or discovering that NVQ or Microsoft Certification courses are available.

Threats: deficiencies in equipment, software or availability of training; other commitments, antagonism or lack of support from others.

You might include a survey of the equipment and software available in your PCG/PCT and elsewhere and list the present competencies of other staff. What levels of expertise are accessible inside and outside your own workplace?

What are the learning needs for the practice and how do they match your needs?
The prioritising exercise should have already given you some information. Consider inviting people to give their concerns and opinions at a practice team meeting or ask another member of staff to organise it. The practice manager could ask people to complete a checklist of their own needs and wishes for IT, and what they would like from others.

One staff member might wish to specialise and become an accredited software or hardware expert. Does that fit with the requirements of the practice (or PCG/PCT)? Would it be more cost-effective to buy in that expertise?

A GP might wish to become the IT adviser for the health authority or the lead for IT in the PCG/PCT. What implications does that have for the practice in terms of cover for clinical sessions?

continued

A secretary may wish to have paid time to go on a computer skills course to learn spreadsheet and database skills. Do you already have someone at a lower grade who can do this or would it free up practice nurse or GP time if she or he took over some of the data management for audits, etc.?

You might discover from the GPs that they would be willing to learn IT skills if they could have a TV card on their PC to watch the cricket, or that providing email or Internet access in the common room would encourage people to use the computers more. This might mean that your needs will be met within the PPDP.

Any patient or public input to your plan?
If you are intending to become 'paperless', what do your patients think about it? Do you know what they think about where the screen is in the consulting room? Do they want to see what you are entering? Have they concerns about who will access the information and the level of confidentiality? How will they be reassured about the collection of data for PCG/PCT management functions?

Do they want to be involved in designing information on health matters? Do they want you to have a website? How do you manage general public enquiries to a practice website? Do they want the development of electronic transmission of prescriptions to the pharmacist of their choice? Do they want to email their prescription requests to you? Would patient-held electronic medical records be acceptable?

If you are introducing an electronic patient call system, take their advice on siting the call boards, the colour of the display, the level of auditory signal, etc.

Discuss the use of computers at the reception desk – are there confidentiality issues that concern patients?

Computer terminals giving access to other sources of advice might be provided by other agencies (libraries, citizens' advice bureau, the Council). What would patients like, and would the general public have access?

Do patients want to use computer programs for health advice or treatment of, for example, psychological problems (cognitive therapy is available as a computer program)?

What mechanism(s) will you use to find out the answers in a meaningful way – not just from the most opinionated or compliant? You may need to think deeply about the reliability of any method and how representative individual patients are of your whole practice population.[3]

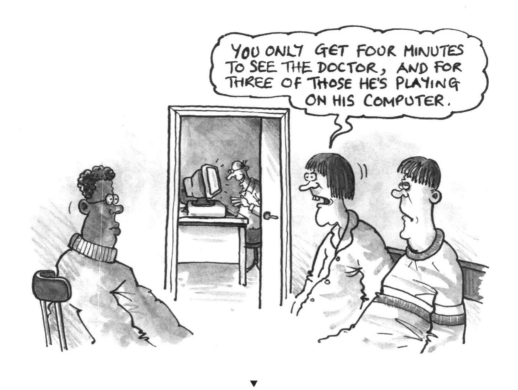

Aims of personal development arising from the preliminary data-gathering exercise

To learn how to, for example:

- use the computer for consulting and prescribing
- set up an appointment and call system and use the system for health promotion messages
- enter Read codes consistently
- do a search and audit and use a spreadsheet
- use email and the Internet
- sort out bugs in the software
- use linking with the health authority and hospital trust for registration, claims and clinical information downloads
- set up forms for automating referrals, management and activity reports, annual report information, etc.
- set up protocols and guidelines for delegation and consistent recording
- use financial management
- produce patient leaflets and a newsletter
- become 'paperless'.

How you might integrate the 14 components of clinical governance into your PDP focusing on the topic of IT

Establishing a learning culture: hold regular meetings on different aspects of IT, including hands-on practice for team members to learn new skills and information.

Managing resources and services: identify whether the computer system is being used to its best capacity, ensuring that service contracts are maintained and are cost-effective.

Establishing a research and development culture: a 'web night', perhaps, to whet people's appetites for searching for health information, using searches to find information, finding out what is being done elsewhere.

Reliable and accurate data: enter data once, enter data consistently and correctly, be able to retrieve it for a variety of uses and be able to compare the data with others.

Evidence-based practice and policy: find out which systems are accredited for use in general practice. Discover the best methods of sending information between computers.

Confidentiality: ensure that passwords are used correctly and securely; that the data is protected against unauthorised access and not passed to others without knowing the degree of confidentiality it will be given. Screens should only be visible to those who need to read them, and information on patients should not be visible to others.

Health gain: more reliable and accessible data means better-quality management and more proactive care, such as call and recall systems.

Coherent team: everyone needs to know how to enter data consistently and to retrieve that part of it that they require for patient management.

Audit and evaluation: check consistent entry of Read codes, follow the management of specific conditions, search and audit care in a multiplicity of ways. Service management can be audited or even your financial management.

Meaningful involvement of patients and the public: use the computer to provide health information requested by patients or to provide an interchange of ideas as in a newsletter written by both patients and staff. Use computer health education or treatment packages, or just use it to provide a randomised stratified selection of patients for your patient focus groups.

Health promotion: target health promotion with specific reminders on screen or select specific groups for action, e.g. to offer smoking cessation.

Risk management: ensure up-to-date records on everything from the patients, to staff qualifications (last cardiopulmonary resuscitation update?) to when the steriliser was last serviced. Reminders for action can be set, interactions of drugs or allergies recorded.

Accountability and performance: your system must have an 'audit trail' to be accredited, i.e. there is a record of who entered what and when. Ensure that everyone knows that they must only log on as themselves and why.

Core requirements: could you work out a better skill-mix in your practice team to provide more cost-effective computer use?

Action plan (include the objectives above, timetabled action, expected outcomes)

Who is involved: all identified staff who need to learn IT skills with you.

Where: identify the sites at which training and learning will take place.

Timetabled action: Start date

By xx month: preliminary data gathered and staff involved identified:

- skills that are already present (in-practice, in the PCG/PCT, health authority, etc.)
- equipment and systems that are available (yours, the practice, the PCG/PCT, outside in a training venue)
- training that can be obtained (to match your needs)
- training that could take place (in-practice, other practice(s), college or university, commercial IT facility, distance learning, other local or distant venue)
- how it could be done (individual or group; tutor led or cascade learning).

By xy month: review current performance:

- are your skills being used in the best way?
- does the equipment meet the specifications for the tasks you are required to perform now and those you anticipate doing in the immediate future?

By yy month: identify solutions and associated learning needs:

- arrange the necessary training
- make a business plan for any associated equipment needs
- arrange cover for yourself and any other staff who are involved to provide protected time for learning
- clarify who does what and when
- negotiate changes necessary at practice meeting(s).

By yz month: make the changes:

- implement the new IT systems or procedures
- obtain feedback from other staff as to its impact
- iron out any difficulties
- identify any gaps in the provision.

Expected outcomes: reliable, accurate data, easily entered and retrieved, ease of use, quicker access to records, better quality of care for patients, better access to care for patients, relevant interdisciplinary shared information, increased safety and security (depending on the exact project carried out).

How does your PDP tie in with your other strategic plans?
(for example the practice's business or development plan, the Primary Care Investment Plan)

Development of IT will be an integral part of your practice business or PPDPs and of your PCG/PCT plans. Make sure that your objectives mesh with theirs.

What additional resources will you require to execute your plan and from where do you hope to obtain them?
Your entitlement to reimbursement of course fees, etc., will depend on your contract and on the priority value that the practice or PCG/PCT puts on your development plan to meet their own needs.
    Any additional equipment will have to be decided on the same basis.

How will you evaluate your learning plan?
Look at the methods you used to identify your learning needs – how does it all fit? Can you repeat a measure that you adopted to establish your learning needs to determine how much you have learnt or the extent to which your performance has improved?

How will you know when you have achieved your objectives?
You will be able to carry out the tasks you have set yourself, or will have implemented the changes specified in your objectives list.

How will you disseminate the learning from the plan to the rest of the practice team and patients? How will you sustain your new found knowledge or skills?
You might let everyone know in a practice newsletter. Let the staff know what has been achieved, or what is now available, at team meetings.
    Pass on your skills to other people in the team as required and keep using your skills to provide information or better structure or systems to your computer programs. You could run an in-house training session to teach others in the practice team how to do one of the new procedures you have mastered.

How will you handle new learning requirements as they crop up?
Keep a record as they arise to consider later or add them in if essential at this stage.

Key facts for IT that you might use to justify the topic as a priority to incorporate in your PDP

- Your local library, medical or otherwise, usually gives assistance about accessing the Internet and using email. Medical libraries can help you learn how to do electronic searches more effectively.
- Other sources are colleges and universities. Contact their IT department. They will usually set up a specific course for your needs if you can recruit several people who want one.
- The journal *Health Service Computing* (available free to doctors and IT professionals working in healthcare from A & M Publishing, First House, Park Street, Guildford, Surrey GU1 4XB or www.hsc.uk.com) is published in association with the RCGP and Cactus – Practice Effective Prescribing and contains useful articles and relevant advertising.
- Most medical computer systems have their own support groups of interested professionals who help the company to develop the software with ideas and testing new programmes. Contact your supplier for details.
- Practical guidance on using the Internet is available from many books. Look at medical ones for more relevant information.[77]
- Medical informatics courses via the Internet are available from several American universities.[78] Included is 'Medical Informatics – a week-long survey course from the National Library of Medicine (home of Medline) designed to familiarise individuals with the application of computer technologies and information science in medicine. A longer course of 11 weeks from Oregon University covers:
  - medical data and its uses
  - evidence-based medicine
  - computer networks
  - telemedicine
  - decision making
  - medical computing
  - information retrieval
  - Internet
  - electronic medical records
  - imaging.
- A report on UK professional qualifications[79] for people working in IT describes a distance-learning course to gain an MSc in health informatics. There is also the NVQ system that non-academic candidates can use to demonstrate their competence by the use of portfolios. This originally resulted in a qualification known as the 'Statement of Recognition' that was refined in 1996 into the practical course resulting in the Diploma or Advanced Diploma in Information and Technology (Health).
- Microsoft Professional Certification can be studied as formal courses with lectures and practical sessions, distance-learning courses or self-paced training. The course

books are available from most large bookshops and computer suppliers. Further information is available from the website (http://www.microsoft.com/mcp).

- The NHS192[80] directory contains details of every UK practice, PCG/PCT and health authority. It is being expanded to include NHS trusts and other organisations throughout the UK. It is likely to save staff a lot of time and trouble. It is available to all NHS staff, including pharmacists, opticians and dentists.
- A smart card for medical records has just been launched. It is initially aimed at people at high risk, such as those with diabetes, epilepsy, heart problems, allergies or special needs. Ambulance crews will be equipped with readers for the smart cards. Gloucestershire, Dudley, Hereford & Worcester, Warwickshire and Bristol are the first areas, before the scheme is extended nationally. Health authorities are being provided with the equipment to read the cards, and subscribers pay a joining fee and a lower annual subscription (£28.50 and £18 respectively at 2000 prices).

Check out whether the topic you choose to learn is a priority and the way in which you plan to learn about it is appropriate

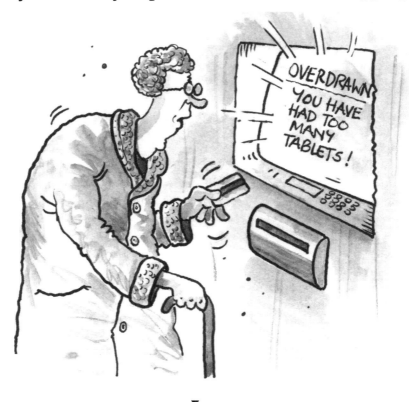

▼
Over-smart cards!

Your topic: information technology

How have you identified your learning need(s)?

a	PCG/PCT requirement	X	e	Appraisal need	❐
b	Practice business plan	X	f	New to post	❐
c	Legal mandatory requirement	❐	g	Individual decision	❐
d	Job requirement	X	h	Patient feedback	❐
			i	Other	❐

Have you discussed or planned your learning needs with anyone else?
Yes   X   No   ❐   If so, who? *Other staff; PCG IT lead*

What are the learning need(s) and/or objective(s) in terms of:
Knowledge: What new information do you hope to gain to help you do this?
To learn how to enter data consistently and reliably and how to retrieve information in a useful form

Skills: What should you be able to do differently as a result of undertaking this learning in your development plan?
Produce the annual report quickly; produce information about workload and services provided by the practice; identify problems with targets at an early stage

Behaviour/professional practice: How will this impact on the way you then do things?
I might be able to improve the quality of information to improve the delivery of services and ensure that all income due for item of service claims is obtained

Details and date of desired development activity: *Within three months: attend sessions on use of the software available on the computer system and Read coding. Within six months: start to produce rolling reports on the services, workload, and targets*

Details of any previous training and/or experience you have in this area/dates:
Piecemeal self-instruction without structure or specific objectives

Your current performance in this area against the requirements of your job:
Need significant development in this area X   Need some development in this area ❐
Satisfactory in this area   ❐   Do well in this area   ❐

Level of job relevance this area has to your role and responsibilities:

Has no relevance to job	❐	Has some relevance	❐
Relevant to job	❐	Very relevant	X
Essential to job	❐		

Describe what aspect of your job and how the proposed education/training is relevant:
Integral part of my work evaluating and monitoring the performance of the practice team

Additional support in identifying a suitable development activity?
Yes   X   No   ☐

What do you need? *To know when and where relevant sessions of training are being held. Help in preparing reports*

Describe the differences or improvements for you, your practice, PCG/PCT or employing NHS trust as a result of undertaking this activity:
I will be able to evaluate the standards of care, monitor performance and assess progress towards targets set by the practice team and PCG. It will be easier to produce the annual report and other information required for outside bodies, e.g. when the practice is assessed

Determine the priority of your proposed educational/training activity:
Urgent   ☐   High   X   Medium   ☐   Low   ☐

Describe how the proposed activity will meet your learning needs rather than any other type of course or training on the topic:
The mix of learning from sessions with an experienced user of the software and personal learning by observing others' practice in different settings should help me identify what I don't know and meet my learning needs

If you had a free choice would you want to learn this? **Yes**/No
If **no**, why not? (please circle all that apply):
waste of time
already done it
not relevant to my work, career goals
other

If **yes**, what reasons are most important to you (put in rank order):
improve my performance   1
increase my knowledge   2
get promotion
just interested
be better than my colleagues
do a more interesting job
be more confident   3
it will help me   4

Record of your learning about IT
You would add the date, length of time spent etc. on each learning activity

	Activity 1: knowledge of best practice in the use of the software	Activity 2: learning skills of Read code and other consistent data entry techniques	Activity 3: learning skills in information retrieval and producing reports	Activity 4: learning how to impart the skills gained to others in the practice
In-house formal learning				Protected time for other practice team members to learn consistent data entry and the reasons for it
External courses	Sessions with experienced users of the computer software	Read coding course; sessions with experienced users in users' group	Attendance at local course on use of Excel and producing reports	A distance-learning course on teaching computer skills
Informal and personal	Sit in with audit clerk, practice manager to discover what their information needs are	Discussion and standardisation agreements with others in the computer users' group and other practices in the PCG	Practice information retrieval and report production	Informal sessions whenever a problem is presented, help offered to others as required, informal discussions about harmonisation of data entry
Qualifications and/or experience gained	Experiences of others at the sessions; gain experience in use	Experience and practice in techniques	Reports produced and available for the practice team and PCG or for outside bodies such as the health authority	Monitoring of data entered and audit of standards

Template for your PDP(complete one chart per topic)

What topic have you chosen?

Who chose it?

Justify why topic is a priority:

A personal or professional priority?

A practice priority?

A district priority?

A national priority?

Who will be included in your personal development plan? (anyone other than you?
– other GPs, employed staff, attached staff, others from outside the practice, patients?)

continued

What baseline information will you collect and how?

How will you identify your learning needs? How will you obtain this and who will do it: self-completion checklists, discussion, appraisal, audit, patient feedback? Look back to the section on identifying your learning needs in Chapter 1.

What are the learning needs for the practice and how do they match your needs?

Any patient or public input to your PDP?

Aims of your PDP arising from the preliminary data-gathering exercise

How might you integrate the 14 components of clinical governance into your personal development plan focusing on the topic of:

Establishing a learning culture:

Managing resources and services:

Establishing a research and development culture:

Reliable and accurate data:

Evidence-based practice and policy:

Confidentiality:

Health gain:

Coherent team:

Audit and evaluation:

Meaningful involvement of patients and the public:

Health promotion:

Risk management:

Accountability and performance:

Core requirements:

Action plan (include objectives, timetabled action, expected outcomes)

How does your personal development plan tie in with your other strategic plans (for example the practice's business or development plan, the Primary Care Investment Plan)?

What additional resources will you require to execute your plan and from where do you hope to obtain them? (will you have to pay any course fees; will you be able to organise any protected time for learning in working hours?)

How will you evaluate your PDP?

How will you know when you have achieved your objectives? (how will you measure success?)

How will you disseminate the learning from your plan to the rest of the practice team and patients? How will you sustain your newfound knowledge or skills?

How will you handle new learning requirements as they crop up?

Key facts about .... that you might use to justify the topic as a priority to incorporate in your PDP

Check out whether the topic you choose to learn is a priority and the way in which you plan to learn about it is appropriate

Your topic:

How have you identified your learning need(s)?

a	PCG/PCT requirement	❑	*e*	Appraisal need	❑
b	Practice business plan	❑	*f*	New to post	❑
c	Legal mandatory requirement	❑	*g*	Individual decision	❑
d	Job requirement	❑	*h*	Patient feedback	❑
			i	Other	❑

Have you discussed or planned your learning needs with anyone else?

Yes ❑   No ❑   If so, who?

....

What are the learning need(s) and/or objective(s) in terms of:

Knowledge: What new information do you hope to gain to help you do this?

....

Skills: What should you be able to do differently as a result of undertaking this development?

....

Behaviour/professional practice: How will this impact on the way you then do things?

....

Details and date of desired development activity:

....

Details of any previous training and/or experience you have in this area/dates:

....

Your current performance in this area against the requirements of your job:

Need significant development in this area	❑	Need some development in this area	❑
Satisfactory in this area	❑	Do well in this area	❑

Level of job relevance this area has to your role and responsibilities:

Has no relevance to job	❑	Has some relevance	❑
Relevant to job	❑	Very relevant	❑
Essential to job	❑		

Describe what aspect of your job and how the proposed education/training is relevant:

....

Additional support in identifying a suitable development activity?
Yes ❑   No ❑

What do you need?

Describe the differences or improvements for you, your practice, PCG/PCT and/or NHS trust as a result of undertaking this activity?

....

Determine the priority of your proposed educational/training activity:
Urgent ❑   High ❑   Medium ❑   Low ❑

Describe how the proposed activity will meet your learning needs rather than any other type of course or training on the topic:

....

If you had a free choice would you want to learn this? **Yes**/No
If **no**, why not? (please circle all that apply):
waste of time
Already done it
not relevant to my work, career goals
other

If **yes**, what reasons are most important to you (put in rank order):
improve my performance
increase my knowledge
get promotion
just interested
be better than my colleagues
do a more interesting job
be more confident
it will help me

Record of your learning:
Write in topic, date, time spent, type of learning

	Activity 1	Activity 2	Activity 3	Activity 4
In-house formal learning				
External courses				
Informal and personal				
Qualifications and/or experience gained				

CHAPTER SEVEN

Integrating your PDP and the PPDP

The practice personal and professional development plan (PPDP) should cater for everyone who works in a practice. Clinical governance principles will balance the development needs of the population, the practice, the PCG/PCT *and* your individual personal development plan (PDP).

You might want to start by identifying your own learning needs, combining them with other people's and then checking them against the practice business plan. You could start from the other direction – develop a practice-based PPDP from your business plan and then identify your individual learning needs within that. Whichever direction you start from, you must ensure that you integrate your individual needs with those of your practice, the wider community, and the needs and directives of the NHS.

Your learning plan should complement the professional development of other individuals and of the practice. If you are working on a project that involves change for other people as well as yourself, it is better to work together towards a common goal and coordinate multiprofessional learning across traditional boundaries.

If you work in a number of different roles or posts, gaps and duplication of activities should be avoided. After reflection about the boundaries between your roles you may be able to focus your learning so that meeting your needs in one role benefits another.

Make your learning plan flexible: you may want to add something in later when circumstances suddenly change or an additional need becomes apparent – perhaps as the result of complaint or hearing something new at a meeting.

Long-term locums (say, longer than six months), assistants, retained doctors and salaried GPs should all be included in the practice plan. Remember to include all those staff who work for the practice, however few their hours – you cannot manage without them or they would not be there!

Time is one of the resources that must be considered when drawing up your action plan. Adequate resources must be in place for your learning needs and protected time must be built in. Gathering adequate funding is usually best done as part of the PPDP by an identified person who can make contact with the clinical governance or education lead of the PCG/PCT about possible sources of help. The new arrangements for funding should encourage coordination and pooling of resources between Education Consortia (for non-medical education, NMET) and the Directors of Postgraduate General Practice Education.[1]

Worked examples

Look back at Chapter 1 to refresh your mind about how you got this far.

This chapter gives five worked examples of PPDPs:

- depression
- back pain
- teenage pregnancy
- diabetes
- coronary heart disease.

The details should give you ideas – they are not intended to be comprehensive and particular pathways will be dependent on your local situation and needs.

The pages of key facts should describe the sort of information and sources of reference that should be useful in justifying that particular topic as a priority issue or as a benchmark against which to compare how your practice fares. For simplicity, we cite publications that carry information about the original references, rather than the specific references themselves.

After the worked examples is a template for you to assess your learning needs as a practice, plan your programme and demonstrate your achievements.

A PPDP focusing on depression

Who chose the topic?

You may have chosen it as a practice team; or there may be one member of the practice staff who champions the topic and gains everyone else's agreement to address it.

Justify why topic is a priority

(i)   A practice and professional priority? Missed depression can mean that the patients concerned are treated for their associated physical symptoms for a considerable time – this may be costly in terms of the quality of patients' lives as well as unnecessary investigations and treatments. If these patients are off work with undetected and untreated depression the social and economic costs to their families are significant.

(ii) A district priority? Yes, many district HImPs have improving mental healthcare as a priority.

(iii) A national priority? Yes 'depression' is a key feature in the NSF on mental health.

continued

Who will be included in the PPDP?

You might include:

- the community psychiatric nurse – practice-attached or NHS trust-employed
- practice nurses
- GPs
- practice manager
- receptionists
- practice secretaries
- community pharmacists
- counsellors – voluntary, Relate, practice-employed
- health visitors
- district nurses
- social workers from local patch
- any interested psychologist or psychiatrist.

Who will collect the baseline information and how?

You might ask for information on the practice population from public health – your practice secretary might send for that. You might run a computer search for medication or other audit of the records – your receptionist or computer operator might do that.

Where are you now? (baseline)

This might include:

- description of practice population – numbers, age, gender; and numbers of patients newly diagnosed with depression in past 12 months. If you cannot retrieve this information in a computerised form, you may have to keep prospective records for three months instead
- comparison of prescribing of different types of antidepressants; between prescribers in your practice; between the practice and other practices. You might receive anonymised PACT data comparing your performance with others from the local prescribing adviser
- referral patterns in past 12 months; to community psychiatric nurse, to counsellors, to psychologists, to practice staff (practice nurse, health visitor), to psychiatrists, to voluntary sector organisations. Compare referral behaviour between practitioners and with other practices. The health authority and hospital trusts may be able to supply you with comparative data
- patient survey – have you undertaken one in relation to depression or about services in general? If so, what did the results show? You might look at satisfaction with explanation, doctor or nurse listening to patient
- audit – did you undertake one recently that would be relevant to 'depression'? If not, you might look at compliance with treatment; such as average length for which patients took medication (e.g. antidepressants) or 'did not attend' figures for referrals to others
- performance indicators held by the health authority or PCG/PCT – do they hold any relevant data on file such as numbers and reasons for complaints?
- numbers and type of staff with relevant expertise in your team. You might map out all those who are practice-team members or to whom you can refer patients – their particular skills and range of help offered. Do you know all the possible sources of help in the voluntary sector and what their qualifications and expertise are?

continued overleaf

What information will you obtain about individual learning wishes and needs?
The prescribing adviser may have visited the practice to discuss your over- or under-prescribing of antidepressants.

A significant event such as where a young man commits suicide should set the team reviewing whether any more might have been done to treat his depression.

The local Mental Health Trust may have unilaterally decided to switch community psychiatric nurses (CPNs) to supporting the 'enduring mentally ill' rather than those patients with mild/moderate depression. You will either have to learn to fight your corner to justify retaining your CPN or redistribute work to the remaining members of the practice team. The latter will create new learning needs for individuals.

You might hold a practice team discussion to elicit people's concerns and their perceptions of the main issues for the practice as individuals and as an organisation. Collect their ideas for solutions. The practice nurse might organise that session.

All members of the practice team might complete a checklist enquiring about their perceived learning needs, and might suggest learning needs other members of the team have (e.g. Dr X does not refer appropriately to the CPN), or how the organisation might be improved (e.g. communication between different members of staff about individual patients is poor). The practice manager might organise that exercise.

The clinicians might be aware that depression is a topic about which they need to learn more as a priority, having discussed it individually with their clinical supervisor (nurse) or educational tutor (GP).

Or you might use other methods of identifying learning needs given in the earlier section of the book, such as by comparing what you do with best practice cited by others.

What are the learning needs for the practice and how do they match the needs of the individual?
Individuals may wish to specialise. For example, the practice nurse may wish to undertake an accredited course on counselling. The nurse's aspirations may match the needs of the practice. For instance, it may be that a practice nurse with more expertise in counselling may replace lost CPN time or meet the needs of a cohort of newly registered refugees housed in your area. But it may be that the practice nurse training would be better targeted at other clinical topics as you already have a sufficient number of trained counsellors among the practice team.

Patient or public input to your plan
You might ask patients with depression about their care, their ideas for improvements and seek feedback on how you are doing.

You might consult your patient panel, if you have one, to ask them for feedback about access and the appointment system, or make suggestions for priority issues you might tackle.

You might include one or two patients who have suffered from depression or their carers to participate in in-house training for staff, to put the patient perspective so that your staff and services become more patient-centred.

How will you prioritise everyone's needs in a fair and open way?
You might gather all the available information and make it available to anyone working in the practice who is interested. You could then decide on the appropriate action at a designated

continued

team meeting where a representative of the nurses, GPs, practice staff and the practice manager attend. The representatives would have talked to other staff members before the meeting so that they could relay their views.

Aims of PPDP arising from the preliminary data-gathering exercise
Aims: to meet the NSF for mental health[81] Standards 2 and 3:

- Standard 2: 'any service user who contacts the primary healthcare team with a common mental health problem (in this case, depression) should have their mental health needs identified and assessed; be offered effective treatments, including referral.'
- Standard 3: 'any individual with a common mental health problem (in this case, depression) should be able to make contact round the clock with the local services (in this case, GPs and the primary care team) necessary to meet their needs and receive adequate care.'

How you might integrate the 14 components of clinical governance into your PPDP focusing on 'depression'

Establishing a learning culture: design the PPDP through a democratic process; involve all relevant professionals (including the community psychiatric nurse and community pharmacist) in practice-based teaching and learning.

Managing resources and services: control how resources for training are allocated according to service relevant needs; alter referral patterns according to agreed practice-based protocol for managing depression.

Establishing a research and development culture: encourage all practice staff to critically appraise the practice protocol and suggest changes to achieve more effective management of depression.

Reliable and accurate data: agree way of recording types of depression to which all staff adhere, e.g. use Read codes; consistent entry on computer for every case seen.

Evidence-based practice and policy: monitor adherence to practice protocol for managing depression; individuals should justify deviation from the practice protocol.

Confidentiality: increase awareness of issues about releasing information about a person's mental health to others, with and without their permission; consider a policy for when patients are so ill and a danger to themselves that it may be ethical to release information without their permission.

Health gain: increase staff awareness of the frequency with which mental ill health presents with physical symptoms; increase staff expertise in detecting new cases of depression.

Coherent team: clearly agree roles and responsibilities in management of depression with everyone working within their areas of competence.

Audit and evaluation: review success of programme to take account of the context and setting as well as clinical expertise and flexibility of practice team to respond to unexpected events such as new model of delivery of care to depressed patients.

continued overleaf

Meaningful involvement of patients and the public: realise that questionnaires are an inappropriate medium for gathering information from people with moderate or severe mental health problems; develop more meaningful methods such as informal interviewing. Involve people with depression in decision making about alternative options for treatment.

Health promotion: screen people for depression – target high-risk groups such as those who have had strokes.

Risk management: anticipate those at risk of attempting suicide and take preventative action whenever possible; reduce missed diagnoses of depression through improved expertise of all staff – clinicians and receptionists.

Accountability and performance: use a mix of the factors in this example to get a more complete picture of your performance.

Core requirements: include time and support for members of the practice team to prevent their becoming depressed or burnt out in response to the volume of work, frequent changes and competing service demands.

Action plan

Who is involved/setting: all staff as set out above

Timetabled action: Start date

By xx month: preliminary data gathering completed and staff involved:

- is there a protocol for managing patients with mild, moderate and severe depression?
- numbers of staff; map expertise completed; list other providers
- referral patterns and prescribing patterns
- information about characteristics of practice population, known performance, local and national priorities
- staff complete checklists giving views and suggestions.

By xy month: review current performance:

- extent of knowledge and usage of practice protocol for managing depression; whether it is it based on best practice and fits with others' management plans (e.g. hospital trust)
- access to appointments, telephone advice – audit of actual performance via pre-agreed criteria
- compare performance with any or several of the 14 components of clinical governance.

By yy month: identify solutions and associated training needs

- set up new systems for appropriate triage of priority patients
- write or revise the practice protocol on the management of depression having searched for other evidence-based protocols; input from practice team and psychiatrist
- agree roles and responsibilities of team for delivering care and services

continued

- apply the protocol, identify gaps in care, and proposed changes to delivery of care or services so that GPs and nurses adhere to protocol
- certain staff attend external courses. Community pharmacist provides some in-house training on prescribing to GPs. Receptionists have in-house training on triage
- liaise with GP Co-operative to review how GP deputies and nurses triage calls from or about those with depression. If there is a widespread learning need contact GP tutor to request series of district-based seminars.

By yz month: make changes

- feedback information to PCG/PCT and NHS trust to justify request for more resources
- improve access, find ways to prioritise patients with depression and other mental health problems; improve security of records and confidentiality of patients' medical details
- community pharmacist help to review repeat prescribing
- increase referrals to voluntary sector
- arrange session from citizens' advice bureau in the practice to help patients claim benefits of which they might otherwise have been unaware
- petition social services and PCG/PCT for practice attached social worker; in the meantime improve access to named social worker at local social services premises.

Expected outcomes: more effective management of depression; better patient compliance with medication and attendance at referrals; more flexible access arrangements; increased help from social services and financial advisers.

How does your PPDP tie in with your other strategic plans?
The management of depression should be a priority for the practice business plan if a great deal of effort is to be expended on improving the care and services of those with depression as described in your practice personal and professional development plan.

What additional resources will you require to execute your plan and from where do you hope to obtain them?
You will require resources for training, and for changing prescribing and referral patterns (this might be an extra cost justified by health gains or cost savings). You will have to readjust current resources or seek additional support from your PCG/PCT; if it is a priority in the district or PCG/PCT's strategic plans, you may be able to tap into any additional resources that are available.

How much protected time will you allocate to staff to undertake the learning described in your plan?
This will depend on your circumstances, aspirations and needs. Staff entitlement to time off or reimbursement of course fees, etc., will depend on their contract and on the priority value that the practice or PCG/PCT puts on their contribution to the development plan.

continued overleaf

How will you evaluate your PPDP? (who will be responsible for what)
You might undertake an audit of any of the aspects of care and services that have featured so far.

You might use a SWOT analysis – but you will have had to anticipate its use in evaluation by undertaking the analysis as a baseline assessment and then reviewing progress at the completion of the initiative.

You might undertake a survey of patient satisfaction or compliance with treatment, before and after your initiative, using patients currently suffering from depression, that is, two separate groups of patients, so long as you have got the first lot better!

How will you know when you have achieved your objectives?
Using the audit and survey methods described above and measuring deviation from the agreed practice protocols.

How will you disseminate the learning from the plan to the rest of the practice team and patients? How will you sustain the new knowledge and skills?
You might write about it in a practice newsletter. Let all the staff know at practice meetings what progress has been made. You might want to talk about your provision at a voluntary group meeting or at a neighbourhood forum. You might want to describe your success at a PCG meeting.

Pass on your skills and knowledge to others as required, review your protocol at set intervals to incorporate new information.

How will you handle new learning requirements as they crop up?
The practice manager who leads the initiative can collate suggestions, complaints, observations as they are made by staff or patients, in response to the new systems. The practice manager and clinical supervisor may revisit the topic of depression in annual appraisals to check on progress and any perceived new learning requirements.

Key facts about depression that you might use to justify the topic as a priority to incorporate in your PPDP

- One quarter of GP consultations are for people with a mental health problem.[81]
- Around 90% of mental healthcare is provided solely by primary care.[81]
- Only about 30–50% of depression in primary care is recognised by GPs.[81]
- One in 15 women and one in 30 men is affected by depression each year.[81]
- A GP can expect to see between 60 and 100 people with depression each year.[81]
- Most of the 4000 suicides in England each year are attributed to depression.[81]
- Rates of depression in people from African-Caribbean, Asian, refugees and asylum seeker communities are around 60% higher than in the 'white' population, in the UK.[81]
- People from black and minority ethnic communities are much less likely to be referred for psychological therapies.[81]
- The government target for mental health is to: 'reduce the death rate from suicide and undetermined injury by at least a fifth by 2010 – saving up to 4000 lives in total'.[81]
- Suicide is more common among those with easy access to killing themselves.[82]
- Many people who are mentally ill die prematurely from physical illness, especially respiratory illness, cancer and coronary heart disease.[81,82]
- The cost per annum of mental illness in England has been estimated to be £32.1 billion.[82]
- Suicide rates in England are equivalent to those in Wales and Northern Ireland and lower than those in Scotland; they are among the lowest in Europe.[82]
- Mental health promotion includes: support from personal relationships, controlling stress from the work environment, relaxation and physical activity. Carers are less likely to be depressed if given practical information about their dependants; unemployed people are less likely to be depressed with social support and help with job seeking skills; immediate help for depressed mothers can prevent adverse effects from their depression being visited upon their children.[82]
- Antidepressant medication is an effective treatment for depression[81]; those shown to be effective long-term include: imipramine, fluoxetine, sertraline, and possibly amitrypyline and maprotiline.[83]
- Older antidepressants are cardiotoxic, dangerous in overdose, and can impair memory and psychomotor function.[83,84]
- Subtherapeutic doses of antidepressant medication are commonly used in general practice.
- Cognitive therapy and interpersonal therapy are as effective as antidepressant drugs 5or mild to moderate depression.[85]
- Problem-solving therapy and St John's Wort are likely to be effective treatments for depression.[85]
- Continuing antidepressant treatment for four to six months after recovery reduces the risk of relapse; maintenance therapy in recurrent depressive disorder reduces the risk of recurrence.[81]

Record of practice team learning about 'depression'
You would add the date, length of time spent, etc. on learning activity

	Activity 1: more rational prescribing	Activity 2: prioritising high-risk patients	Activity 3: awareness of non-NHS helping agencies	Activity 4: revise practice protocol on management of depression
In-house formal learning	Health authority prescribing adviser held a small group session to review prescribing patterns of each GP partner, and compare the practice with others	Practice team event to which practice manager and GP presented update on depression – signs and symptoms, risk management, and ideas on systems and procedures to improve access		Final practice protocol described and explained at practice team event (see Activity 2). All roles and responsibilities of GPs, nurses, receptionists and practice manager agreed
External courses	Prescribing was one topic in day's update course on 'depression' at local postgraduate centre			GPs and practice nurse attended day's update course on depression
Informal and personal	Two GPs read up on the topic and worked together to review prescribing in the practice protocol on the management of depression. Practice nurse joins in online discussion group debating best practice	Practice nurse stuck newspaper cutting up on staff room noticeboard of 'traffic light' system used on medical records of patients known to be at high risk in another practice	Manager of citizens' advice bureau, officer from MIND and Relate counsellor all visit practice for half an hour at coffee time to meet staff informally and tell team members about their services	GP, practice nurse and practice manager drafted practice protocol in preparation for other team members to comment on it
Qualifications and/or experience gained		Practice manager visited other practice in PCT to see how receptionists spot high-risk patients and arrange urgent access there	One practice nurse decides to train to be a Relate counsellor as a 'volunteer'	

A PPDP focusing on back pain

What topic?
Back pain: in relation to (i) looking after backs of practice staff (ii) patients consulting with back pain.

Who chose topic?
The practice manager might suggest focusing on it from a 'good employer' angle. The clinical staff (GPs and nurses) might recognise that updating their management of back care is a key need for them too when the physiotherapist asks them to be more explicit in their referrals so that he or she can prioritise urgent cases and they are uncertain of what constitutes 'urgent' criteria.

Justify why topic is a priority

(i)   A practice and professional priority? Preventing back problems from manual handling by practice staff should reduce sickness absence; arranging that referrals for X-rays are undertaken at an appropriate time for patients with significant back problems should ensure that patients are not exposed to unnecessary risks from radiation.

(ii) A district priority? Reducing the numbers of inappropriate back X-rays by GPs with the highest referral rates should reduce costs.

(iii) A national priority? The government has a national *Back in Work* initiative that aims to reduce sickness absence from back problems among the workforce.[86] Appropriate early management of acute back pain will reduce the development of long-term, chronic back pain.

Who will be included in the PPDP?
You might include:

*   GPs
*   practice nurses
*   district nurses
*   practice manager
*   receptionists
*   practice secretary
*   cleaners
*   community pharmacists
*   community physiotherapist
*   local osteopath
*   chiropodist/podiatrist
*   chiropractor
*   patients.

Who will collect the baseline information and how?
You might ask the local X-ray department to supply quarterly data of your referrals. A baseline audit by one of the receptionists might look at how often the occupation was recorded in patients' records for those suffering from back pain. The practice manager might keep a

continued overleaf

prospective record of any staff member experiencing backache triggered or made worse by work. The practice manager or community physiotherapist could review the practice environment and watch people in their everyday work looking for causes of any back problems that could be remedied.

Where are you now? (baseline)
This might include:

(i) Good employer practices – back problems in staff
*   Is there a policy for minimising back problems in staff as part of an overall policy on health and safety/occupational care of staff? Are any measures in place to prevent back pain in staff: for example, has there been a training session on manual handling for all practice staff (including the cleaners) in the past two years and who attended? Have sources of back problems for staff been reviewed (such as awkward filing cabinets; difficulties of getting heavy or disabled patients on to examination couches); and if so have measures been taken to minimise potential sources of back problems?
*   Are there any special sources of advice and help for staff with back problems: for example, special ergonomically designed chairs, literature, fast-track to a physiotherapist?

(ii) Clinical management
*   Whether the practice has a protocol or guidelines for best practice in managing back pain or problems. If not, a description of what GPs believe to be their usual practice for patients with differing degrees of back pain over time.
*   Whether the GPs and nurses in the practice know of providers of alternative medicine, such as osteopaths, herbalists, aromatherapists, acupuncturists, chiropractors, homeopaths or remedial therapists, and refer patients to them and are familiar with their qualifications, range of therapies, the likely evidence for the alternative therapies, availability and cost, etc.
*   Audits of aspects of clinical management: for example, numbers of patients prescribed anti-inflammatory drugs for back pain, number X-rayed, number receiving magnetic resonance scan (MRI), numbers referred to NHS physiotherapy and for orthopaedic opinions from hospital consultants. You might compare your clinical management with others.
*   Whether GPs and nurses and pharmacists promote exercise for all patients, especially those with back problems; is there an exercise referral scheme to local leisure centres – is it used? Do the practice staff know what leisure services are available locally?
*   Potential range of provision of therapeutic and investigative services available to clinicians.

What information will you obtain about individual learning wishes and needs?
You might hold a practice team meeting and invite members to describe any causes of back problems for them.

   You may undertake a significant event audit after one of the district nurses hurts her back while on a home visit, lifting a patient who had fallen on the floor. Or you might have had a critical incident where a patient who was on anti-inflammatory drugs for back pain had a sudden fatal haematemesis. A district-wide audit of the numbers of X-ray investigations of

continued

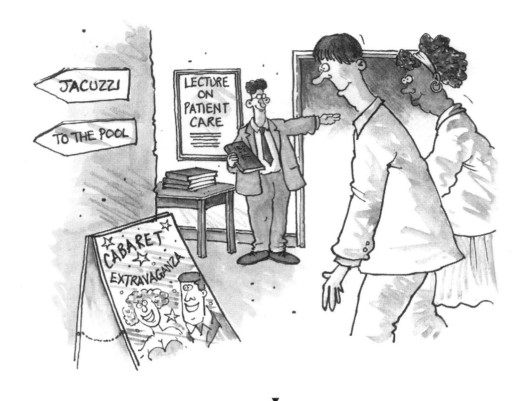

▼

the lumbo-sacral spine might reveal whether your practice makes comparatively more or less referrals than other similar practices.

You could undertake an audit of the next 20 consecutive patients who have had back pain for at least three months to see how their experiences tally with how you expect your services to operate. You might find that there was a reason why they did not access your care before, if this is their first visit. You may find that they have not been advised to stay active or that they ignored such advice and went to bed (this might reveal learning needs – not being able to convince the patients of recommended practice).

Or you might use other ways of identifying learning needs given in Chapter 1 – looking at adherence and deviation from practice protocols, reviewing learning needs that have arisen from job appraisals (e.g. those of the cleaners), looking at whether the extent of staff care (e.g. preventing causes of back problems) matches the standards expressed in your practice or PCG/PCT strategies.

What are the learning needs for the practice and how do they match the needs of the individual?

The practice manager is the obvious person to take lead responsibility for ensuring that the practice improves the way it operates to prevent back problems in staff or minimise the

continued overleaf

effects of back problems if staff are back pain sufferers. So the practice manager would have to ensure that staff were trained in manual handling and knew about back care. The practice manager would need to involve the GPs. The GPs would need to understand the importance of investing in equipment and office furniture to minimise the risk of back problems occurring, and join in any training on learning to lift in a trouble-free fashion or avoid lifting heavy weights altogether.

The GPs, nurses and pharmacist could draw up a protocol or guidelines for the practice based on recommended best practice in back care management; or adopt recommendations from elsewhere. If current practice is demonstrated to be putting patients at unnecessary risk by over-investigation by X-rays, giving inappropriate medication, or costing the patients avoidable time off work, then everyone should agree to adhere to the PPDP, even if not particularly eager to learn more about managing back pain.

Patient or public input to your plan
You might hold an open evening to which most of the practice staff contribute short talks or demonstrations of best practice in back care. A physiotherapist or osteopath might show people how to lift heavy objects, do back strengthening exercises and maintain good posture; a spokesman from leisure services might describe their equipment; a GP or chiropractor might talk about what people with back pain can do for themselves. A podiatrist might stress the importance of good footwear to correct an abnormal gait.

You might ask patients with back pain to tell you how you might improve your services (for instance by making a back support available at reception to ease discomfort sitting on the surgery chairs if those with back problems have a long wait to see the doctor).

How will you prioritise everyone's needs in a fair and open way?
You will have to prioritise spending on training and equipment, probably allocating these according to who is in most need – because they are most exposed to triggers of back pain or already suffer from back problems themselves.

An audit of individuals' performance might indicate which of the clinicians are most in need of updating. If one individual takes a lead in finding out how best practice in back care might be instituted in the practice, then resources for education and training (time and money) might be spent on them. Then they can cascade their learning in-house to the other members of the practice team.

Aims of the PPDP arising from the preliminary data-gathering exercise
To meet the objectives of the *Back in Work* initiative:

- 'To reduce the misery and cost of back pain to those in the workplace'[86]: (i) in your practice; (ii) to patients in general.
- 'To promote good practice in back care management within a framework that includes prevention, assessment, treatment and rehabilitation'.[86]

How you might integrate the 14 components of clinical governance into your PPDP focusing on 'back pain'

Establishing a learning culture: the community physiotherapist might facilitate a meeting where you consider how back problems arise from working in the practice or during home visiting. This topic is common to everyone, whether they are a cleaner, member of the ancillary staff, manager, nurse or doctor. It might therefore be a good topic to draw a multidisciplinary group together and start off regular educational meetings in the practice.

Managing resources and services: preventing back pain and problems in the staff should reduce sickness absence.

Establishing a research and development culture: key messages that have arisen from research have been that exercise and normal daily activities shorten the length of the episode and hasten a return to work when compared to rest; and that X-rays of the lumbar spine are inappropriate for short-lived episodes. Incorporating these recommendations into everyday practice should demonstrate to practitioners how research can be applied in practice and make an impact on the quality of patient care.

Reliable and accurate data: collect information about cases of back pain seen (numbers, location, severity, length of episode, referrals, etc.) and monitor adherence to practice protocols such as appropriate referrals for X-rays.

Evidence-based practice and policy: knowing the evidence for all types of therapies from conventional NHS care to a range of alternative therapies will help the doctor or nurse to make a balanced judgement about referral to an appropriate therapist; or explain the options to patients in an informed way.

Confidentiality: the consulting patient should feel that information from their medical records will be shared on a need-to-know basis with other health professionals. In any audit or research study, access to patients' medical records should be controlled and limited, with informed consent from the patients concerned and ethical approval of the study protocol if necessary.

Health gain: reduction in numbers of inappropriate X-rays will lessen the risk of adverse effects from unnecessary exposure to radiation. Early and effective interventions will get people back to normal activities as soon as possible.

Coherent team: more understanding of the roles and capabilities of therapists should result in a more coherent plan of management and more effective teamwork.

Audit and evaluation: audit any aspect of management, such as numbers and timing of referrals, promotion of normal activities and non-compliance, and make recommendations for evidence-based practice.

Meaningful involvement of patients and the public: consult people in your patient population with and without back problems about which alternative therapies should be available as part of the NHS.

Health promotion: exercise promotion will be a mainstay of management by all clinicians, whether doctors, nurses or therapists.

Risk management: good risk management should reduce causes of back pain for staff working in the practice and avoid or minimise likely causes of work-related back pain.

Accountability and performance: more teamworking will require everyone to be clear about their roles and responsibilities in back pain management.

Core requirements: adherence to current recommended best practice should be cost-effective with savings from reduction in inappropriate referrals for investigations, less time off work and earlier interventions by therapists.

Action plan

Agree who is involved/setting: as staff set out previously – specify names, posts.

Timetabled action: Start date

By xx month: preliminary data gathering and baseline of providers completed:

- is there a protocol for managing patients with mild, moderate and severe, acute and chronic back pain?
- numbers of staff; map expertise; list other providers
- referral patterns to X-ray, orthopaedic consultant, physiotherapy; prescribing patterns
- information about characteristics of those recorded on practice computer as having experienced back pain
- any relevant local and national priorities; and any additional associated resources that might be applied for
- staff discussion to report problems that might trigger back pain, views and suggestions
- practice manager reviews surgery and observes people at work to detect potential sources of back problems.

By xy month: review current performance:

- level of knowledge and use of practice protocol or guide for managing back problems; extent to which protocol or guide fits with best practice or others' back care management plans (e.g. hospital trust)
- audit of actual performance via pre-agreed criteria, e.g. with respect to referrals, promotion of exercise and normal activities
- compare performance with any or several of the 14 components of clinical governance, for example managing resources and services.

By yy month: identify solutions and associated training needs:

- set up new systems for appropriate referral and management
- give receptionists in-house training in manual handling
- revise the practice protocol on the management of back problems/pain as a practice team, with input from physiotherapist, to address identified gaps in care, having undertaken search for other evidence-based protocols. Agree roles and responsibilities as a team for delivering care and services according to protocol; certain staff attend external courses. Community pharmacist, health promotion facilitator and physiotherapist provide some in-house training to GPs and nurses
- order new office furniture as necessary.

By yz month: make changes

- clinicians adhere to practice protocol – as shown by repeat audit of increased/decreased referrals to X-ray, therapist, orthopaedic consultant as appropriate
- practice staff lift less heavy/awkward loads in better style
- back pain sufferers take more exercise and pursue normal activities whether they are practice staff or patients.

Expected outcomes: more effective management of back pain; better patient compliance with exercise and attendance at referrals; less sickness absence due to back pain.

How does your PPDP tie in with your other strategic plans?

Looking after staff's backs and wellbeing should tie in with the practice policy for good employer practices. The initiative should tie in with the PCG/PCT's policy to provide better occupational healthcare of staff and reduce sickness absence of the NHS workforce.

What additional resources will you require?

You should draw up a statement that explains your policy for subsidising or covering the cost of staff course fees. Then everyone knows where they stand when they apply to undertake a course and how the 'rules' for reimbursement vary according to whether the course is entirely to meet the individual's needs or the practice's or NHS requirements.

You are likely to buy replacement office furniture and to fund that from the practice.

Changes in referral patterns are likely as a result of learning activities – to reduce referral activity or divert referrals to less 'expensive' providers such as physiotherapists rather than orthopaedic consultants.

How much protected time will you allocate to staff to undertake the learning described in your plan?

That will depend on your circumstances, aspirations and needs. Staff entitlement to time off or reimbursement of course fees, etc., will depend on their contract and on the priority value that the practice or PCG/PCT puts on their contribution to the development plan.

How will you evaluate your learning plan?

You might re-audit any of the aspects of care and services that have featured so far.

You might undertake a survey of staff satisfaction with the new office furniture and their back comfort, before and after your initiative.

How will you know when you have achieved your objectives?

Use the audit and survey methods described above and measure deviation from the agreed practice protocol.

Compare numbers of patients referred for exercise promotion, physiotherapy and X-ray investigation at baseline with those rates 12 months later.

Record whether staff from different disciplines have taken part in the initiative, attended training on manual handling and put that learning into practice when lifting.

How will you disseminate the learning from the plan to the rest of the practice team and patients? How will you sustain the new knowledge and skills?

You might write about it in a practice newsletter. Let all the staff know at practice meetings what progress has been made. You might want to talk about your provision at a community group meeting or at a neighbourhood forum. You might want to describe your success at a PCG meeting.

Pass on your skills and knowledge to others as required, review your protocol at set intervals to incorporate new information.

How will you handle new learning requirements as they crop up?

Undertake an audit of the next significant event to find out whether the preceding care and services adhered to the practice protocol. If not, determine why not; and if so, what else should be changed or learnt?

Key facts about back pain that you might use to justify the topic as a priority to incorporate in your PPDP

- About 7% of the adult population in the UK present to their GP with back pain in any one year.[87]
- An estimated 19 deaths may arise from the 700 000 people in the UK who have lumbar spine radiographs each year.[88]
- Two in every five adults in the UK report suffering from back pain lasting more than one day in the previous 12 months. Of the people who reported back pain, one sixth said they were in pain throughout the year, and a third described back pain as having restricted their activities in the previous month.[89]
- 5% of back pain sufferers had taken time off work in the previous month according to a national survey.[89]
- Once a person has been off work with back pain for six months, they have about a 50% chance of getting back to work.
- It is estimated that back pain accounts for about 100 million lost working days per year in the UK and around £500 million in health and welfare costs.[88]
- Around 30% of episodes of acute back pain result in persistent disabling symptoms.[90]
- Continuing ordinary everyday activities leads to the most speedy recovery and least time off work; a planned return to normal work within a short time, leads to less time off work in the long run.[91]
- Non-steroidal anti-inflammatory drugs prescribed at regular intervals give effective pain relief in simple acute backache.[90]
- Muscle relaxant drugs are effective in reducing back pain.[91]
- Psychosocial factors influence response to treatment and rehabilitation.[91]
- Manipulation provides short-term improvement in pain and activity for acute and subacute back pain; risks of complications are low.[91]
- Ice, heat, short-wave diathermy, massage and ultrasound help symptom relief but do not appear to speed recovery.[91]
- Transcutaneous electrical nerve stimulation (TENS) relieves symptoms rather than influences the speed of recovery.[87]
- Exercise programmes can improve pain and functioning in people with chronic low back pain.[91]
- Antidepressant medications are widely used for chronic low back pain.[91]
- Acupuncture may reduce pain and increase activity in people with chronic back pain.[91]

Record of practice team learning about 'back pain'
You would add the date, length of time spent, etc. on learning activity

	Activity 1: avoiding back problems in the practice	Activity 2: best practice in the management of back pain	Activity 3:	Activity 4:
In-house formal learning	Physiotherapist ran 'how to lift' session for GPs, nurses and non-clinical staff	Local radiologist, orthopaedic consultant, community physiotherapist contribute to 'roadshow' held in practice for patients and staff		
External courses	Practice manager attended update seminar on health and safety that included latest legislation	GPs attend lunchtime lecture about best practice in the management of back pain		
Informal and personal	Practice nurse and practice manager accompanied physiotherapist and patient round the surgery looking at potential triggers of back problems in surgery environment	GPs chat with staff and practice manager in the course of the week about advantages of introducing an exercise prescription referral scheme. GPs swap tips with other GPs at lunchtime lecture		
Qualifications and/or experience gained	Practice manager gained a certificate of attendance at the health and safety seminar	One GP registers for medical acupuncture course to extend range of treatments that the practice can offer		

A PPDP focusing on reducing teenage pregnancy

Who chose topic?

A GP or practice nurse may be disheartened by yet another youngster with an unplanned pregnancy. The practice team as a whole may choose the topic having been shocked by the magnitude of the local problem when the public health department circulates statistics on numbers of teenage pregnancies, live births and terminations, in the district.

Justify why topic is a priority

(i)   A practice and professional priority? You may have had teenagers present late with a concealed pregnancy too scared to come forward for help any earlier; you might have a batch of young people consulting too late for emergency contraceptive tablets. The local family planning clinic might be closing to save funds and you realise that the practice must absorb the additional work as a consequence.

(ii   A district priority? The rates in your district might be higher than average (see key facts). But as rates in the UK are higher than those in Europe, even the districts with the lowest rates in the UK cannot afford to be complacent.

(iii)   A national priority? Yes, reducing teenage pregnancy is a national priority led from the Social Exclusion Unit (*see* key facts).

Who will be included in the practice-based plan?

You might include:

* GPs
* practice nurses
* health visitors
* social workers – local ones
* community pharmacist
* receptionist
* practice manager
* clinical medical officers and nurses from local family planning clinic
* school nurses
* schoolteachers, head teachers, chair of parent–teacher association
* community development workers who work with young people in locality
* officer of relevant local voluntary organisation
* young people and parents.

Who will collect the baseline information and how?

You might ask your local public health department to keep you updated on teenage pregnancy rates in your district. The local teenage pregnancy coordinator or the sexual health coordinator for your district (probably based in your local health promotion department or public health department of your health authority) should be able to supply information about available services and resources and local projects.

continued

Set up a prospective record of numbers of young women becoming pregnant under 20 years old in your practice population and the outcomes of their pregnancies.

Where are you now? (baseline)

This might include:

- The number of pregnancies in age bands: under 16 year olds; 16- and 17-year-olds; 18- and 19-year-olds. You may plan different tactics to make an impact on pregnancy rates in each age band.
- The number of women of all ages taking emergency contraception and time taken after unprotected sex: tablets and intrauterine contraceptive devices (IUCDs).
- How often boys and young men come for contraceptive advice and supplies (if you can distribute condoms) on their own or with their girlfriends.
- The services that exist in your locality for providing contraception, and any dedicated to serving young people. Judge how convenient the timing and frequency of your services in the practice and the local family planning clinics are. Consider how accessible clinics are for young people without transport who may be closely watched by their parents. Find out if there are school nurse drop-in clinics inside or outside school premises and where and when they are.
- The services that exist in the locality for advising young people about risk taking in respect of their lifestyle – in the NHS, education and voluntary sector.
- Extent to which GPs and nurses in your practice are trained in family planning matters. How many can advise on and fit IUCDs, are up to date with the latest ways of providing emergency contraception, understand the barriers that obstruct young people from seeking contraceptive advice and supplies, and are aware of the importance of counselling and teaching about relationships as well as providing contraceptives?
- Measures you take in the practice to be flexible to young people's requirements, and overcome young people's apprehension and reluctance to consult. Measures you take to be proactive, such as invitations to young people to come for health checks and counselling.
- Extent of sex education locally, including whether any NHS staff are involved in the delivery of school- or college-based teaching or help, e.g. school nurses.
- Any resources that are available to help any future initiative, such as whether you can tap into a condom distribution scheme, or contribute to a local radio campaign.
- Extent of literature or educational material you have about contraception for young people – is it suitable or dated?

What information will you obtain about individual learning wishes and needs?
You might hold a practice team meeting to discuss the problem – the receptionists might describe what happens when a young person rings up or comes in at inconvenient times when no GP or nurse is free or on the premises. The GP and nurse might discuss the most recent advances in emergency contraception. Others present may realise that they need to know more and request that the practice manager arranges a more comprehensive educational programme and suggest how it might be conducted.

continued overleaf

You might undertake an audit of a significant event such as of a 15-year-old who presents with a 30-week pregnancy; try to find out where and when anyone might have intervened to have avoided a pregnancy or encouraged the girl to have presented earlier. A GP or practice nurse or community midwife could do this from the notes, by talking to the girl, her parents and any health professional who had seen her within the previous four months (taking care to adhere to good practice in preserving confidentiality).

You could compare the GPs' rates of prescribing of emergency contraceptive pills with those in other practices; deducing that there may be a problem of access to services or knowledge/skills of GPs if your practice has a lower-than-average rate (although this might be because you have proportionately less young girls in your practice population or are located near to an accessible family planning clinic).

Or you might use other methods of identifying learning needs given in the earlier section of the book – from job and educational appraisals, reading and reflecting, or comparing your own practice with a best practice model cited from elsewhere, for example.

What are the learning needs for the practice and how do they match the needs of the individual?

The practice manager should take responsibility for reviewing the accessibility and convenience of services for young people. He or she may have to learn how to be more responsive to young people's needs. The receptionists will probably need training on how to be more accommodating to young people amidst the hurly-burly of a busy practice.

The practice nurse or a GP might take responsibility for agreeing a practice protocol for providing up-to-date emergency contraceptive services for those of all ages seeking help after unprotected sex. Or compare the guideline describing the standard practice response to under-16-year-olds seeking contraception, covering the roles of the receptionists, nurses and GPs. Each stage in the protocol or guideline will have associated learning needs for those unsure of their responsibilities or unprepared for their roles.

The practice manager, and possibly a GP who takes an educational lead for the practice, might weigh requests from individuals for further training in this topic with the needs of the rest of the practice team, as demonstrated by the preliminary work done so far, then take a strategic approach to furthering the skills of the practice team as a whole. It is likely that everyone will need more training on understanding young people's needs and constraints and this might be a good topic for an in-house training session to which everyone working in the practice or attached to it, is invited.

Patient or public input to your plan

You won't get very far with improving the services your practice provides if you don't know what young people themselves want, and hear their views. You might ask young people for their views as they attend, or while you are building up a close relationship with them providing antenatal care. You could go to the local school and contribute to a pastoral lesson about relationships and listen to their concerns and issues.

You might invite a parent of a young person who has had an unplanned pregnancy to join your in-house training session; or even a 16- or 17-year-old who has had a recent unplanned pregnancy might feel confident enough to join you.

continued

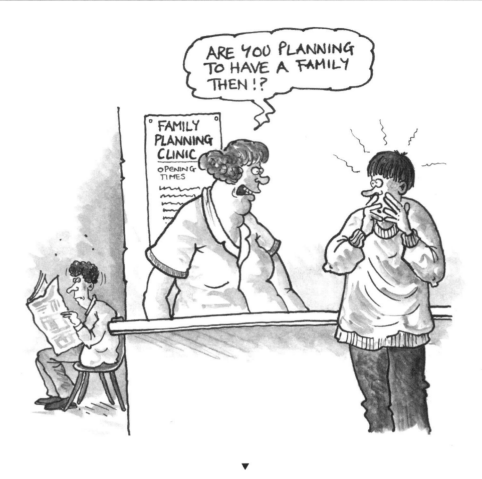

How will you prioritise everyone's needs in a fair and open way?

You might set up your own working group on reducing teenage pregnancy in your practice if the problem is significant enough. A GP, school nurse, practice manager and receptionist might form a group that undertakes a baseline review of the scale of the problem, available services and resources, individuals' learning needs and others' strategies, then listens to the other members of the practice team and outside agencies before planning changes to services and arranging staff training.

Aims of PPDP arising from the preliminary data-gathering exercise

To contribute to the objectives of the Social Exclusion Unit:[92]

- to reduce the rate of teenage pregnancies, specifically to halve teenage pregnancies by 2010
- to prevent the causes of teenage pregnancy – which from a primary care perspective is to provide accessible and flexible contraceptive services to young people that include counselling about the risks of unprotected sex.

How you might integrate the 14 components of clinical governance into your PPDP focusing on the topic of teenage pregnancy

Establishing a learning culture: multidisciplinary working should include: the receptionists being flexible when responding to young people's requests for help, doctors being up to date on the latest emergency contraception, practice nurses acquiring more insight into young men's needs and counselling about personal relationships.

Managing resources and services: plan which skills you need and equip your workforce with those skills.

Establishing a research and development culture: find out what young people want, how best to engage them and make an impact on their behaviour. Search the literature for examples of best practice. Should you undertake your own study?

Reliable and accurate data: know how many young people are attending for contraception and whether there are clusters of unplanned pregnancies in particular areas. Improve your data recording and plan who will be involved in this.

Evidence-based practice and policy: a clinical update meeting might focus on the 'best' ways to explain risk to young people. Incorporate the evidence into improved ways of working.

Confidentiality: everyone should know and understand the rules for preserving confidentiality in under-16-year-olds.

Health gain: there are direct health gains for the young person, their parents and the unborn child, e.g. avoiding poverty, low birth weight babies. Include learning about the wider determinants of health in your plan.

Coherent team: partnership working will lead to those in the NHS working more closely with anti-poverty workers in the city council, social workers working with children in care, education – schools and general public, the media and press. You have to create and sustain partnerships – plan for how to do that.

Audit and evaluation: monitor how many young people consult for contraception. Plan and execute improvements in services and the associated learning.

Meaningful involvement of patients and the public: improve staff expertise in engaging individual young people in making decisions and informed choices. Seek input or exchange information about the services you provide. If you do not know much about meaningful involvement, incorporate that learning into your plan.

Health promotion: learn more about the subsequent effects of sexual infection – increased rates of infertility from infection with *Chlamydia*. Learn about the association of alcohol and drug misuse with unwanted pregnancy and how to motivate teenagers to resist or reduce risky behaviour.

Risk management: concentrate on learning to control risk – lack of continuity of care, poor communication, informing virgins about emergency contraception; work with teachers and parents to give them accurate information about contraception; debunk myths that might tempt young people to take a risk.

Accountability and performance: demonstrate the standards of services you provide and the care for which you are accountable; evaluate your performance and any changes.

Core requirements: deliver education and training in-house and through external courses so that your staff are competent and their skill-mix suits your local circumstances.

Action plan (include objectives, timetabled action, expected outcomes)

Agree who is involved/setting: as staff set out previously – specify names, posts.

Timetabled action: Start date

By xx month: preliminary data gathering and completion of baseline of providers:

- is there a practice protocol or guide on accommodating young people wishing to access services, providing emergency contraception, etc?
- numbers of staff; map expertise; list other providers
- referral patterns for terminations, antenatal care
- information about characteristics of those recorded on practice computer as having a teenage pregnancy
- any relevant local and national priorities; and any additional associated resources for which you might apply
- staff discussion to report problems that limit young people accessing services, observed problems, views and suggestions.

By xy month: review current performance:

- practice manager reviews operation of services and closeness of working relationships with those in other organisations and sectors who have an interest or responsibility for young people's education and welfare
- clinical lead reviews extent of knowledge and skills of practice team with respect to routine contraception for young people, emergency contraception, handling young people
- audit of actual performance via pre-agreed criteria, e.g. with respect to referrals, sexual health promotion, contraceptive prescription and compliance
- compare performance with any or several of the 14 components of clinical governance, for example confidentiality would be very relevant.

By yy month: identify solutions and associated training needs:

- set up new systems for access to contraceptive services appropriate to young people's needs
- give practice team in-house training on dealing with young people
- revise the practice protocol on provision of routine and emergency contraception to address identified gaps in care, having undertaken search for other evidence-based protocols. Agree roles and responsibilities as a team for delivering care and services according to protocol; certain staff attend external courses. Practice or school nurse or GP provide some in-house training to other GPs and nurses, community pharmacist or others from outside organisations with whom practice is liaising over the issue.

By yz month: make changes:

- clinicians adhere to practice protocol – as shown by repeat audit of experiences of those young people who have an unplanned pregnancy
- change to service times and locations that are more appropriate for young people; organise training to anticipate new requirements, e.g. train community pharmacist to be able to counsel and supply emergency contraceptive pills.

Expected outcomes: more effective prevention of unplanned pregnancy in general and in teenagers in particular; fewer sexual diseases; better compliance with contraception.

How does your PPDP tie in with your other strategic plans?
Your educational programme should tie in with similar initiatives in other practices, in the PCG/PCT, across the district and in schools and other young people's settings. The district's teenage pregnancy coordinator will cite your practice team as an example of best practice if your learning plan is comprehensive and tied into your practice development.

What additional resources will you require to execute your plan and from where do you hope to obtain them?
This will depend on your circumstances, aspirations and needs. Staff entitlement to time off or reimbursement of course fees, etc., will depend on their contract and on the priority value that the practice or PCG/PCT puts on their contribution to the development plan.

How will you evaluate your learning plan?
You might re-audit any of the aspects of care that have featured so far.
    You might ask a couple of young people who consult for contraceptive purposes to report their experiences back to you. The practice team should have previously agreed the exercise but not know when or who will observe and report on their systems and procedures.

How will you know when you have achieved your objectives?
Monitor the levels of teenage pregnancies. Look at numbers of young people consulting at the practice and local clinics with sexual diseases.

How will you disseminate the learning from the plan to the rest of the practice team and patients? How will you sustain the new knowledge and skills?
You might write about it in a practice newsletter. Let all the staff know at practice meetings what progress has been made. You might want to describe your success at a PCG meeting.
    Pass on your skills and knowledge to others as required, review your protocol at set intervals to incorporate new information.

How will you handle new learning requirements as they crop up?
Ask the working group who are leading the practice initiative to reduce teenage pregnancies to note down learning needs they observe in the rest of the team or that are reported to them by patients or staff members. These may be fed into your current PPDPs or inform next year's plans.

Key facts about teenage pregnancy that you might use to justify the topic as a priority to incorporate in your PPDP

- The problem: 90 000 teenage girls pregnant each year in England; 56 000 give birth.[92]
- 7700 under-16-year-old girls in England become pregnant each year.[92]
- Pregnancy rate per 1000 girls aged 13–15 years = 8.8 in England and Wales; there are regional variations between 6.6 in Anglia and Oxford to 10.5 in the West Midlands region with wide variation between local authority areas, e.g. 20.4 in Lambeth to 4.4 in Barnet (Clinical and Health Outcomes Knowledge Base (July 1999) National Centre for Health Outcomes Dept).
- Terminations: half under-16s and more than one third of 16s and 17s opt for a termination.[92]
- 15 000 under-18-year-olds have a termination per year in England.[92]
- About one third of under-16-year-olds are sexually active.[92]
- Teenagers are susceptible to sexual infection – 1% get HIV, 30% herpes, 50% gonorrhoea after a single episode of unprotected sex with an infected partner.[92]
- The death rate of babies of teenage mothers is 60%, higher than for babies of older mothers.[92]
- Teenage pregnancy is more common if young people have had disadvantaged childhoods and have low expectations of education or a job.[92]
- Teenage pregnancy is associated with an increased risk of poor social, economic and health outcomes for both mother and child.[93]
- School-based sex education does not increase sexual activity or pregnancy rates.[93]
- Increasing the availability of contraceptive services for young people is associated with reduced pregnancy rates.[93]
- Young people do not travel easily; they want services at a central location with discreet premises that are easy to find. Drop-in services should be available during the lunch hour, late afternoon or early evening.[30]
- You should reorientate existing services so that they are acceptable, accessible and appropriate to a wide range of young people.
- Prevention programmes should be targeted at vulnerable groups and local contexts.[94]
- Prevention programmes should reinforce value messages such as saying 'no'.[94]
- Staff working with young people should provide a non-judgemental service.
- Vulnerable groups include: non-school attendees, young people who are the off-spring of young parents, homeless or run-away children, teenagers living in deprived areas, young people in care ('looked-after children').[94,95]

Record of practice team learning about 'reducing teenage pregnancy'
You would add the date, length of time spent, etc. on learning activity

	Activity 1: understanding young peoples' perspectives and needs	Activity 2: knowledge of scale of problem: local teenage pregnancy rates	Activity 3: best practice in offering contraception to young people	Activity 4: know whereabouts and type of contraceptive services for young people in locality
In-house formal learning	Training session run by local youth worker on understanding young peoples' needs and constraints; all practice and attached staff attended		Practice team meeting where roles and responsibilities are agreed around a practice protocol; GP who is also a family planning clinic doctor facilitates learning	School nurse describes drop-in clinics, where and when they are, to practice manager who cascades information. Practice nurse designs newssheet with this information for young people
External courses		Hour session at local university on epidemiology attended by GP on Masters in Health Policy	All GPs and nurses in the practice who are not trained in family planning and who provide contraceptive services attend course	
Informal and personal	GPs, nurses and practice manager listen to audio tape on this topic while driving in their cars	Circular from local public health department of teenage pregnancy rates in your district – discussed and debated by GPs and practice nurses over coffee	Reading, reflecting on and learning new recommendations for emergency contraception through individual study	
Qualifications and/or experience gained			Family Planning Certificate – newly acquired or updated through continuing education	

A PPDP focusing on diabetes mellitus

Who chose topic?
Many of the practice team may realise that improving the care of patients with diabetes is of overriding importance after the preliminary learning needs assessment described in Chapter 1, or the district or PCG/PCT may be undertaking a strategic review of diabetes and their questions to the practice may uncover many weaknesses in the current diabetes care and services.

Justify why topic is a priority

(i) A practice and professional priority? Good risk management is an essential part of diabetic care at a clinical level for individuals with diabetes, and from an organisational perspective in identifying new cases and monitoring their continuing care. So investing time and effort in improving the care of those with diabetes should produce tangible and significant health gains for individual patients.

(ii) A district priority? Many districts have set up diabetic registers and have local initiatives to improve the management of those with diabetes and more 'seamless' care across the primary/secondary care interface.

(iii) A national priority? The cost of medical complications in diabetic patients is high. Effective diabetic management is cost-effective to the NHS, through avoiding complications, keeps those with diabetes at work as well as maintaining their health and wellbeing. Diabetes is a national priority being the subject of a NSF.

Who will be included in the practice-based personal and professional development plan?
You might include:

- GPs
- practice nurses
- health visitors
- district nurses
- diabetic liaison nurse from local NHS trust
- optometrist
- community pharmacist
- chiropodist or podiatrist
- practice manager
- reception staff
- British Diabetic Association representative
- patients with diabetes, and their families.

Who will collect the baseline information and how?
A receptionist/computer operator could do an electronic search in your practice to identify those with diabetes if appropriately coded. Otherwise it will be laborious setting up a diabetic

continued overleaf

disease register from paper records, repeat prescriptions, recall, etc. Once you know who your diabetic patients are, you can audit their care and see what you need to learn.

The local public health department at your health authority should be able to supply data about morbidity and mortality rates in your district. They may also have national data on file about the average numbers per 1000 population who might be expected to have diabetes broken down by age, gender and ethnic group; or you can obtain this information from your local medical library.

The local hospital trust could give you routine and acute data about referrals and admissions of those with diabetes. The hospital audit department may have undertaken work on diabetes and might give you a breakdown of results identifying your patient or PCG/PCT populations.

Where are you now? (baseline)

- Establish how many diabetics you have, and whether they are insulin-dependent, on oral hypoglycaemic drugs or controlled by diet; by age groups.
- Compare your practice protocol for managing diabetes with a protocol cited in the literature as 'best practice' or a recommended district protocol or guideline. If you do not have a practice protocol write one or adopt someone else's.
- Look at how many attend follow-up appointments in line with your practice protocol – for the various groups with diabetes, different age groups or ethnic groups. Deduce whether you may need to make follow-up appointments more available or convenient.
- Determine how good glucose control is in your patients with diabetes. How many have good control with an HBA1c $< 6.5\%$; how many are borderline at HBA1c 6.5–7.5%; how many have poor control $> 7.5\%$?
- Focus on prevention of risks, such as looking at numbers who smoke or are overweight; or assess the quantity and quality of literature available for patients in your practice.
- Review the extent of education or training the clinical staff have had about diabetes.

What information will you obtain about individual learning wishes and needs?
You might review the practice protocol and baseline information with as many staff as possible at a discussion group and find our whether they feel competent as individuals to carry out their roles and responsibilities, or want to realign their duties. They might comment on how well others are fulfilling their responsibilities and suggest improvements to the systems or procedures that have educational and resource consequences – training sessions, new equipment, effects on other parts of the practice organisation.

A significant event audit, such as if a person with diabetes becomes blind or has a leg amputated, or someone aged under 60 years old with diabetes has a myocardial infarction, might reveal learning needs of individuals and practice systems.

You might develop a checklist from the self-appraisal included on pages 9–10 in Chapter 1 for individual members of staff to indicate their perceived needs.

What are the learning needs for the practice and how do they match the needs of the individual?
Compare your own figures for numbers of people with diabetes with those you would expect in a practice population of your size and demographic make-up. Conclude whether you need

continued

to be more proactive in identifying new cases of diabetes; and address lack of knowledge or skills, uncaring attitudes or inadequate systems.

Compare prescribing patterns featuring in current PACT data between the GPs in your practice, and with other practices, to look for differences and inconsistencies that might indicate learning needs.

A patient complaint from the parents of a 10-year-old boy about the delay in detecting his diabetes may reveal learning needs for particular individuals or the practice organisation.

Compare your practice protocol for the management of diabetes with other 'gold standard' protocols or recommended guidelines (*see* Key facts) to reveal learning needs. These may be educating patients, counselling about the implications and consequences of diabetes, monitoring, self-management and pharmacological treatment with insulin or oral antidiabetic agents to achieve specific glycaemic goals.

Undertaking a SWOT analysis as a practice team (*see* Chapter 1) in response to the queries from the district or PCG/PCT about the practice's diabetic services might reveal inadequacies in your baseline knowledge of what services you are providing, how they are used or what you are achieving. You should include the employed and attached staff as well as independent contractors, such as the local optometrist and community pharmacist.

A staff member, such as the practice nurse or health visitor, might have nominated diabetes as a topic they wished to learn more about at their annual job appraisal. If no one else in the practice has expert knowledge or skills in the management of diabetes, then it will be well worth the practice facilitating the nurse to attend an in-depth course.

The practice manager may be new to the area and intend to visit other practices to learn the ropes; she or he might take a particular interest in observing how other practices run their services for those with diabetes. This focus might justify additional time spent on practice visiting.

Patient or public input to your plan

Ask the parents who made the complaint to help you devise better systems in the practice or write an account of their experiences that can be used for an in-house training session.

You might ask the local representative of the British Diabetic Association or a patient with diabetes to attend an informal training session – in particular dealing with educating and informing patients better, motivating patients about prevention of risks, side effects of treatment.

An open evening on diabetes that is held for those with diabetes and their families will provide an opportunity for patients to mix with GPs, nurses, therapists, optometrists and non-clinical staff; informal conversations during the evening should reveal learning needs and ideas for improvements.

Aims of PPDP arising from the preliminary data-gathering exercise

After gathering baseline data and undertaking a preliminary learning needs assessment you might design a PPDP that has a grand, overarching aim: to develop a learning programme for all members of the practice team, attached staff and independent contractors (such as optometrists and community pharmacists) to enable them to provide effective management of diabetes within available resources.

continued overleaf

Or you might concentrate on developing particular key individuals, e.g. a GP or practice nurse or specific receptionist with lead responsibility for the clinical management or practice organisation of diabetes. They could then cascade their learning in-house to others in the practice team.

Or you could focus down on aspects of the effective management of diabetes. For instance: to develop a learning programme for all members of the wider primary healthcare team to increase their knowledge and skills in educating and informing patients and their families about good practice in the management of diabetes. This might include learning how to motivate patients to comply with recommended management practices, avoid risks and complications, comply with treatment.

How you might integrate the 14 components of clinical governance into your PPDP focusing on 'diabetes'

Establishing a learning culture: a multidisciplinary team might update their learning about reducing cardiovascular risks in non-insulin dependent diabetic patients. The practice manager could learn about providing services that are more sensitive to detecting new cases of diabetes, facilitate attendance for follow-up care and encourage compliance. The nurses and GPs could learn about risk management and better ways to motivate patients to achieve satisfactory glycaemic control.

Managing resources and services: promote close working relationships and teamwork between the practice-employed staff, independent contractors such as the optometrists and trust-employed staff such as podiatrists.

Establishing a research and development culture: encourage practice team members to critically appraise published papers describing new findings in diabetic care, to check out whether the results described are applicable to their population.

Reliable and accurate data: keep good records to enable active follow-up of any patients with diabetes who are unable to get to the surgery such as the housebound, or others who fail to attend at regular intervals.

Evidence-based practice and policy: the practice protocol for people with different types of diabetes should be based on the best evidence for the population and local circumstances.

Confidentiality: there should be water-tight systems to prevent any information about a patient having diabetes being released without their express permission. Any issues of confidentiality should be clarified before information about individual patients is passed to a district register of diabetic people.

Health gain: good glycaemic control reduces the risk of complications from diabetes.

Coherent team: all the practice team should understand the roles that the attached podiatrist, optometrist and pharmacist play in providing and monitoring care, and reducing the risks of complications.

Audit and evaluation: a significant event audit of, for example, a person with diabetes becoming blind should indicate areas where further training is required, or practice services and teamwork should be improved.

continued

Meaningful involvement of patients and the public: a roadshow demonstrating good diabetic care held in the surgery and attended by representatives from the voluntary sector, patients, clinicians and support staff should engage people with diabetes and their families. A focus group of diabetic patients might reveal shortcomings in staff knowledge and attitudes or malfunctioning practice systems.

Health promotion: it is essential that people with diabetes do not smoke as this escalates their risk of cardiovascular complications. The practice staff should target diabetic patients with advice about their lifestyle.

Risk management: identify and control risks as the bedrock of the management of diabetes, to reduce the likelihood of complications.

Accountability and performance: demonstrate that the advice and treatment staff are providing to people with diabetes is in line with best practice.

Core requirements: practice staff should be competent and trained for the roles and responsibilities that are delegated to them by the GPs and practice manager.

Action plan (include objectives, timetabled action, expected outcomes)

Agree who is involved/setting: as staff set out previously – specify names, posts.

Timetabled action: Start date

By xx month: preliminary data gathering and collation of baseline of providers:

- is there a practice protocol or guide on effective management of diabetes?
- numbers of staff; map expertise; list other providers
- referral patterns for routine advice and monitoring of diabetes, admissions, for advice/help for complications
- information about characteristics of those recorded on the practice computer as having diabetes – age groups, ethnic origins
- any relevant local and national priorities; and any additional associated resources for which you might apply
- staff discussion to report problems that limit those with diabetes of different age groups, etc., accessing services, observed problems, views and suggestions.

By xy month: review current performance:

- practice manager reviews operation of services and closeness of working relationships with those in other organisations and sectors who have an interest or responsibility for diabetes
- clinical leads (e.g. GP, nurse) review extent of knowledge, skills and attitudes of practice team with respect to routine care of those with diabetes of all types
- audit actual performance versus pre-agreed criteria, e.g. with respect to referrals, education given to those with diabetes, investigations, monitoring and compliance
- compare performance with any or several of the 14 components of clinical governance, for example health promotion would be very relevant.

continued overleaf

By yy month: identify solutions and associated training needs:

- set up new systems for access to services appropriate to needs of those with diabetes
- give practice team in-house training on important aspects of managing those with diabetes
- revise the practice protocol. Address identified gaps in care, having undertaken search for other evidence-based protocols. Agree roles and responsibilities as a team for delivering care and services according to protocol; certain staff attend external courses. Practice or district nurse, GP, podiatrist or optometrist provide some in-house training to other GPs and nurses, community pharmacist or others from outside organisations with whom practice is liaising over the issue.

By yz month: make changes:

- clinicians adhere to practice protocol – as shown by repeat audits; patient feedback
- change service times and locations so that they are more appropriate for diabetic patients of various age ranges and ethnic groups, having organised training to anticipate new requirements, e.g. train podiatrist to fit with other members of primary care team in surgery setting.

Expected outcomes: more effective prevention of diabetic complications; better patient compliance with treatment and good lifestyle habits; tighter glucose control; fewer of those with diabetes lost to follow-up.

How does your PPDP tie in with your other strategic plans?
The practice's business plan and the PCG/PCT's Primary Care Investment Plan might both prioritise achieving more effective management of diabetes. The PPDP that focuses on diabetes would complement those strategic plans.

What additional resources will you require to execute your plan and from where do you hope to obtain them?
The practice might pay for the course fees of any member of staff undertaking training that fulfils a priority need of the practice.

You may be able to justify an application for additional resources to your PCG/PCT or health authority or local NHS trust with your preliminary learning and health needs assessments, tapping into the district or national strategic priorities.

If a member of staff is undertaking the training on behalf of the practice you should try to arrange for the training to be undertaken in paid time. Any learning cascaded to other members of the practice team as part of the PPDP should also be undertaken in paid time and during working hours whenever possible.

continued

How will you evaluate your PPDP?

You should be able to pick out methods of evaluation from the range of methods suggested for assessing learning needs in Chapter 1. The most appropriate methods will depend on what specific aims you set for your PPDP; for example if your main aim is to achieve the best possible glucose control of people with diabetes, you might evaluate this by monitoring HBA1c levels. But if your aim was to improve the levels and appropriateness of education and information for people with diabetes, you might evaluate your achievements by asking the patients themselves – by a simple test of knowledge, focus group discussion of experiences, monitoring changes in patient behaviour, etc.

The practice manager and clinical lead for diabetes (e.g. GP or practice nurse) might plan the evaluation together and delegate the collection of data to a receptionist.

How will you know when you have achieved your objectives?

Usually this will be by comparing outcomes of your programme with baseline data. But it might be also determined by looking at patients' compliance with recommended practice, or their levels of self-confidence in managing their diabetic condition; asking and attending for help at appropriate times.

How will you disseminate the learning from the plan to the rest of the practice team and patients? How will you sustain the new knowledge and skills?

You might write about it in a practice newsletter. Let all the staff know at practice meetings what progress has been made. You might want to describe your success at a PCG meeting.

Pass on your skills and knowledge to others as required, review your protocol at set intervals to incorporate new information.

How will you handle new learning requirements as they crop up?

The practice manager might run audits at intervals and feed the results back to a practice meeting mid-way through the time period of the PPDP when there is time to revise the activities.

Key facts about diabetes that you might use to justify the topic as a priority to incorporate in your PPDP

- Diabetes occurs in around 5% of adults aged 20 years or over.[96]
- Over a million people in the UK have diabetes; the majority have Type II diabetes.[84]
- Long-term complications of diabetes are: retinopathy (and blindness), nephropathy (and renal failure), peripheral neuropathy (and foot ulcers, amputation), autonomic neuropathy (and gastrointestinal, sexual and bladder dysfunction) and large-vessel atheroma (and myocardial infarction, stroke, peripheral vascular disease).
- Diabetic retinopathy is the most common cause of blindness in people of working age in industrialised countries. Up to 40% of Type II diabetics have some retinopathy when diabetes is first diagnosed.[84]
- It is thought that comprehensive screening and treatment for diabetic retinopathy could prevent 260 new cases of blindness in the UK every year.[84]
- Diabetes is characterised by fasting glucose $\geqslant 7.0$ mmol/l, or two-hour post-75 g oral glucose load plasma glucose $\geqslant 11.1$ mmol/l on two or more occasions.[84]
- Diabetes mellitus increases the risk of cardiovascular disease.[96] Cardiovascular risk factors in diabetic patients include: age, prior cardiovascular disease, cigarette smoking, hypertension, dyslipidaemia, sedentary lifestyle, family history of premature cardiovascular disease, elevated urinary protein excretion, poor glycaemic control.
- Aggressive control of hypertension in people with diabetes (target blood pressures 130/80–85 mmHg or lower) reduces cardiovascular morbidity and mortality.[96]
- Aspirin is effective in primary and secondary prevention of cardiovascular disease in people with diabetes and dyslipidaemia.[96]
- Cigarette smoking increases the risk of cardiovascular death in people with diabetes up to fourfold depending on the amount smoked.[96]
- Screening and referring people with diabetes with altered sensation in feet and absent pedal pulses (i.e. they are at high risk of developing foot ulcers) to footcare clinics (for education, footwear and podiatry) reduces risks of foot ulcers and major amputation.[96]
- 15% of people with diabetes develop foot ulcers associated with neuropathy and ischaemia. Serious infection originating in a diabetic ulcer is the most common reason for amputation, apart from trauma.[84]
- People most likely to develop diabetes include: the obese, people of Asian, African or African-Caribbean origin, people aged over 65 years, those with a family history of diabetes or cardiovascular disease, women with a history of gestational diabetes or who have given birth to a baby weighing > 4 kg.[84]
- There is 'strong evidence' that intensive glucose control reduces the development and progression of microvascular and neuropathic complications in Type I and Type II diabetes, compared with conventional treatment.[97]

Record of practice team learning about 'diabetes'
You would add the date, length of time spent etc. on learning activity

	Activity 1: revise practice protocol	*Activity 2: update patient education*	*Activity 3: identification of new diabetics*	*Activity 4: preventing complications of diabetes*
In-house formal learning	Practice team discussion around roles and responsibilities of various members to fulfil protocol, including podiatrist and optometrist	A pharmaceutical representative shows a non-promotional video on educating people with diabetes watched by GPs and nurses and community pharmacist	GP and nurse with new ideas on targeting and detecting (*see below*) share ideas with rest of practice team during practice discussion of diabetic protocol (*see Activity 1*)	Hospital specialist input to follow-up practice team discussion when changes to practice protocol are reviewed; with any changes in HBA1c levels resulting
External courses	GP lead on diabetes attends two-day continuing medical education course on diabetes at regional centre			Practice nurse attends half-day course on health promotion and motivating patients; she extrapolates this learning to diabetes
Informal and personal	Practice nurse searches for examples of best practice on Medline at home. Practice manager rings up other practices to ask other practice managers if they have protocols and discuss differences	After watching video, practice manager brings in all diabetic literature and audio-visual aids available. Team sorts according to criteria already set from a previous initiative on asthma	GP attending two-day external course and practice nurse attending local practice nurse group meeting pick up tips for targeted screening and being more alert to possibility of diabetes	Practice team members all learn from talking to patients with diabetes in course of daily work how to make more impact with recommendations for a healthier lifestyle
Qualifications and/or experience gained	GP receives accreditation for two-day course that can be put towards a university certificate in health practice			Practice nurse attendance at half-day course is recorded in her own reflective portfolio for discussion with clinical supervisor

A PPDP focusing on coronary heart disease

Who chose topic?

The practice team chose it as a result of undertaking a significant event audit after the unexpected death of Sid, a 45-year-old, from a myocardial infarction. The practice team agreed that coronary heart disease (CHD) should be a main topic in their PPDP as there seemed to be so much they needed to learn.

Justify why topic is a priority

(i)   A practice priority? The practice team were horrified to find out that they had never measured Sid's blood pressure nor checked his cholesterol despite his having a family history of heart disease, and being seen three times in the six months preceding his death.

(ii)   A district priority? The practice team were aware that CHD was a local priority in the district's HImP. The district has higher morbidity and mortality rates for CHD than other comparable areas in the UK.

(iii)   A national priority? CHD is a national priority being the subject of a NSF. The purpose of the NSF is to drive up quality, tackle variations and inequalities in CHD care and services, between different subgroups of the population and between areas.

Who will be included in the practice personal and professional development plan?

- GPs
- practice nurses
- practice manager
- receptionists
- district nurses
- community pharmacists
- health visitors
- public and patients.

Who will collect the baseline information and how?

The practice manager might collect background information about current performance, others' perspectives, options for standards and guidelines they might adopt, available resources and sources of additional resources for the future.

Where possible information could be requested from the primary care development manager of the PCG/PCT acting as a central resource of the information available within the PCG/PCT. The practice manager might organise receptionists and the practice secretary to help with the data collection.

Where are you now? (baseline)

The topic of CHD might include management of angina, myocardial infarction, hypertension, screening for and control of cholesterol.

continued

You as a practice might collect information about:

- all relevant recent practice-based initiatives: suggestions from patients/staff, minutes of practice meetings in past 12 months
- any recent audit of the extent of aspirin taking by those for whom it is clinically warranted with respect to their history of CHD
- PCG/PCT's workforce plan describing how the practice's workforce numbers compare with their peers
- objectives of PCG/PCT's primary care investment plan
- practice-based prescribing data on statins, hypertensive drugs, aspirin
- the health profile of the local community, local morbidity and mortality rates from the health authority – compare any practice-specific data with district figures
- the HImP and other relevant district health reports and strategies – how relevant do they seem to your circumstances? What can you learn from them to help you in your everyday work?
- any health needs survey already undertaken by the local authority concerning lifestyle
- information from local voluntary groups about how available they think services are in your practice; and their suggestions for improvements
- minutes of meetings of local community health forums – see if there is any mention of CHD matters
- district guidelines on referrals to the cardiology directorate – can you compare your referral patterns with those advised?
- published guidelines about managing cardiac conditions and hypertension – compare your practice protocols and see if you can justify any variations.

What information will you obtain about individual learning wishes and needs?
The practice manager might talk to representatives of the practice team individually about the demands of their posts, priorities, roles and responsibilities. All the team could complete checklists describing their:

- roles and responsibilities
- own learning needs
- comments on other team members' learning needs
- ideas on what their standards of CHD care should be
- their personal aspirations and visions for the practice.

The practice manager could then collate this material and discuss it with the GP in the practice who leads on educational matters and the practice nurse who is responsible for clinical governance. They might commission another case-note audit on hypertension, comparing your performance as a practice with that described in their preferred guidelines.

You might use any of the other methods for identifying and assessing learning needs as described in Chapter 1 such as observing how other practices do it. Could one of the practice nurses or receptionists do an exchange with a member of staff in another practice?

continued overleaf

What are the learning needs for the practice and how do they match the needs of the individual?

The practice might prioritise learning according to the requirements of the Standards in the NSF on CHD, relevant to the primary care setting.

Any individual staff members who put themselves forward to learn more about any of these particular topics are likely to find that their learning can be prioritised if the practice is weak in that area, such as how to undertake an intervention or motivate patients to do so, how to apply audit in practice, introducing more effective management of CHD as a whole or one of the conditions coming within the umbrella of CHD. This might be a practice nurse learning more about smoking cessation, a GP attending an update on the prescribing of statins, or a secretary learning more about efficient ways of managing practice disease registers.

Patient or public input to your plan

You might target patients who do not attend or who do not comply with recommended treatment and find out why by asking them directly.

You might set up a patient panel within your adult practice population; randomly select 30 patients from your practice list. Write to them and invite them to participate as either occasional face-to-face meetings or a quarterly postal survey. Ask them whether you have got your services right; if they are convenient, accessible and appropriate. Pose questions relevant to CHD.

How will you prioritise everyone's needs in a fair and open way?

A practice meeting might be devoted to:

- discussing and sorting all the information about performance
- the team members' views about possible improvements
- the importance of the learning needs that have been identified
- the priorities for practice
- considering the impact of the PCG/PCT's plans
- the practice circumstances, aspirations and plans for changes to services.

Then a 'Hanging Committee' of a GP, nurse and practice manager could be convened to prioritise the educational plan for the practice focused on CHD, as described in Chapter 1.

Aims of PPDP arising from the preliminary data-gathering exercise

To develop a learning programme that underpins the achievement of milestones within the Standards of the NSF on CHD. For example to:

- incorporate evidence-based interventions for the secondary prevention of CHD
- achieve the various milestones within the Standards, such as maintaining good records
- establish and maintain and use a register of patients with CHD
- undertake clinical audit
- adhere to a locally agreed protocol on assessment, treatment and follow-up of CHD patients.

How you might integrate the 14 components of clinical governance into your PPDP focusing on 'CHD'

Establishing a learning culture: review the application of the practice protocol for responding to a myocardial infarction; this should involve all the practice staff in multidisciplinary learning about their roles and responsibilities – from the receptionist who recognises the urgency and arranges ambulance transport, to the GP who decides whether he or she can reach the patient before the ambulance to provide aspirin, pain relief and a defibrillator, and to ensure that all staff are up to date with cardiopulmonary resuscitation training.

Managing resources and services: equipment should be regularly checked and in good order, e.g. sphygmomanometers, defibrillator, emergency bag with relevant drugs.

Establishing a research and development culture: investigate whether there are any differences between the levels of treatment and investigation between men and women or different ethnic groups that are not accounted for by the severity of their conditions.

Reliable and accurate data: establish a reliable way of identifying patients with CHD and an accurate way of classifying their condition and cataloguing their tests so that you can offer patients the most effective preventive treatment and monitor their response.

Evidence-based practice and policy: cite the evidence for prescribing statins if your drug budget is inflated according to recommended guidelines for best practice.

Confidentiality: patients should give informed permission before being subjected to any activities outside usual NHS practice, such as taking part in any research study into the treatment or management of CHD, or being videoed for educational purposes.

Health gain: CHD is one condition where there is a great deal of evidence about how many lives are saved by using effective treatments. This is often described as the numbers needed to treat (NNT) with a specific intervention giving a beneficial health gain.

Coherent team: good teamwork is essential for managing patients with CHD where many different disciplines, clinical and non-clinical staff all play a part in prevention and the various stages of acute and chronic treatment.

Audit and evaluation: audit whether prescribing is rational and consistent, whether patients comply with treatment and advice, numbers of smokers, etc.

Meaningful involvement of patients and the public: hold an open evening in the practice around the theme of CHD where you not only give patients as a whole more information about preventing CHD and effective management, but also invite patient feedback about your services. Act on this feedback for it to be 'meaningful' and make changes to your practice's systems and services as appropriate.

Health promotion: smoking cessation, reductions of salt and weight – all decrease risks of CHD.

Risk management: reduce the risks of individuals with CHD by more effective prevention and management; or reduce the risks of a mistake or omission in a practice service by introducing tighter procedures or better monitoring systems.

Accountability and performance: with the good teamwork involving a wide range of staff from different disciplines all playing their part, comes the need for clear lines of accountability.

Core requirements: secondary prevention with statins should be a cost-effective option in that you should save on the costs of secondary care cardiac services and save human lives.

Action plan (include objectives, timetabled action, expected outcomes)

Agree who is involved/setting: as for staff set out previously – specify names, posts.

Timetabled action: Start date

By xx month: preliminary data gathering and collation of baseline of providers:

- are there practice protocols for the management of the various components of CHD – angina, post-myocardial infarction, hypertension, screening for and control of cholesterol, smoking cessation, etc?
- numbers of staff; map expertise; list other providers
- referral patterns for CHD conditions – acute admissions and routine
- information about characteristics of those recorded on practice computer as having CHD – including breakdown by gender, age, co-existing conditions such as diabetes
- any relevant local and national priorities; and any additional associated resources for which you might apply
- staff report problems that limit people accessing services, observed problems, views and suggestions.

By xy month: review current performance:

- practice manager reviews operation of services and closeness of working relationships with those in other organisations and sectors who have an interest or responsibility for CHD, e.g. cardiac rehabilitation
- clinical lead reviews extent of knowledge and skills of practice team with respect to routine care of all aspects of CHD
- audit actual performance versus pre-agreed criteria, e.g. with respect to referrals, health promotion, management, investigation and compliance
- compare performance with any or several of the 14 components of clinical governance, for example clinical risk management would be very relevant.

By yy month: identify solutions and associated training needs:

- set up new systems for access to services appropriate to people's needs
- give practice team in-house training on dealing with those with various conditions grouped under umbrella of CHD
- revise the practice protocol on provision of routine and emergency management to address identified gaps in care, having undertaken search for other evidence-based protocols. Agree roles and responsibilities as a team for delivering care and services according to protocol; certain staff attend external courses. Practice nurse or GP provides some in-house training to other GPs and nurses, community pharmacist or others from outside organisations with whom practice is liaising over the issues.

By yz month: make changes:

- clinicians adhere to practice protocol – as shown by repeat audits
- change service times and locations to ones that are more appropriate for people with CHD or who are being screened for risk factors. Organise training to anticipate new requirements, e.g. train practice nurse about detecting and controlling risks of CHD.

Expected outcomes: more effective prevention of CHD in general; better compliance with treatment and healthy lifestyle advice, revised practice protocols for the management of hypertension, control of hyperlipidaemia, ultimately lives saved.

How your PPDP ties in with your other strategic plans
CHD might be a key item in the annual priority-setting exercise for the practice business plan. The extent of education and development needed would be revealed by the preliminary needs assessment, the high CHD mortality and morbidity rates of the local population, and the realisation that the practice should invest in two new defibrillators for the doctor on call and for the practice treatment room.

The PPDP that focuses on CHD will tie in with the NSF on CHD and subsidiary local initiatives.

What additional resources will you require to execute your plan and from where do you hope to obtain them?
The practice might pay for the course fees of any member of staff undertaking training that fulfils a priority need of the practice.

You may be able to justify an application for additional resources to your PCG/PCT or health authority or local NHS trust based on your preliminary learning and health needs assessments, tapping into the district or national strategic priorities.

If a member of staff is undertaking the training on behalf of the practice you should try to arrange for the training to be undertaken in paid time. Any learning cascaded to other members of the practice team as part of the PPDP should also be undertaken in paid time and during working hours whenever possible.

How will you evaluate your PPDP?
Exact evaluation activities will depend on the aims and content of the learning plan. The practice might re-audit their management of hypertension, hyperlipidaemia and post-myocardial infarction a year after setting out on the plan.

A SWOT analysis undertaken as part of the preliminary needs assessment will lend itself to being reviewed once the learning plan is in place or completed, to note changes that have occurred and the extent to which 'weaknesses' have been redressed and 'threats' minimised.

Other techniques described in assessing and identifying learning needs in the first section of the book might be used for evaluation too, such as observation of practice, review of achievements during subsequent educational or job appraisals, or a repeat computer search to check developments with CHD register.

How will you know when you have achieved your objectives?
Usually this will be by comparing outcomes of your programme with baseline data. You should undertake your evaluation so as to be able to demonstrate the extent to which you have met the milestones within the Standards of the NSF on CHD.

How will you disseminate the learning from your plan and sustain the developments and newfound knowledge or skills?
A member of the practice might attend the local community forum where health matters and community safety are always on the agenda, to give and receive information relating to CHD among other health issues.

continued overleaf

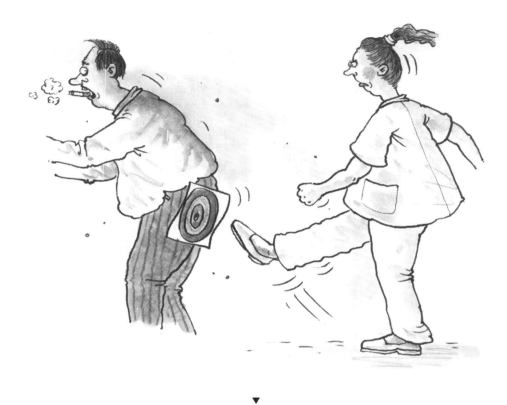

▼
Target health promotion on high-risk groups.

A practice awayday would provide a good opportunity to share learning and plan how to reorganise the practice team to provide more effective care of patients with CHD. Then arrange training for those who require additional knowledge and skills to fulfil their new roles and responsibilities for the intended altered methods of working.

How will you handle new learning requirements as they crop up?
The practice manager might run audits at intervals and feed the results back to a practice meeting mid-way through the time period of the PPDP when there is time to revise the activities.

Key facts about CHD (including angina, myocardial infarction, hypertension, screening for and control of cholesterol)

- Restricting sodium intake and losing weight can result in reducing blood pressure; non-pharmacological interventions can be effective.[98]
- Consider other methods of reducing the risk of CHD before prescribing statins – advice and help on stopping smoking, dietary advice to lower weight and lipids, advice on regular physical activity, control of hypertension, aspirin therapy if appropriate.[84]
- A practice with a 15 000 practice population brought its prescribing of statins in line with the Standard Medical Advisory Clinic (SMAC) guidelines[84] for secondary prevention and increased prescribing of statins from 9 to 103 patients.[99]
- Prescribe statins to those who have had a heart attack and have total cholesterol of 4.8 mmol/l or more, or have angina and total cholesterol of 5.5 mmol/l or more.[84]
- Consider prescribing statins to people without symptoms of CHD who have a high cholesterol and at least a 3% risk per year of a major coronary event.[84]
- The most effective form of cardiac rehabilitation is a combination of exercise, psychological and educational interventions.[84]
- All patients with symptomatic heart failure and evidence of impaired left ventricular function should be treated with an angiotensin-converting enzyme (ACE) inhibitor.[84]
- Treatment of heart failure with ACE inhibitors is cost-effective.
- Patients who have had a myocardial infarction, have had a stroke or transient ischaemic attack and those with stable and unstable angina should all take 75 mg aspirin daily.[84]
- Patients with a suspected acute myocardial infarction should take 150 mg aspirin daily and continue that dose for one month when the diagnosis is proven.[84]
- Local guidelines for responding to patients with a possible myocardial infarction should ensure prompt access to a defibrillator; relief of pain and anxiety.[84]
- All adults should have their blood pressure measured routinely at least every five years until the age of 80 years unless they have high normal values (135–139/ 85–89 mmHg), when blood pressure should be remeasured annually.
- Drug therapy for hypertension should be started in all patients with sustained systolic blood pressure > 160 mmHg or sustained diastolic blood pressure > 100 mmHg despite taking non-pharmacological measures.[84]
- Drug therapy is indicated in patients with sustained systolic blood pressures of 140–159 mmHg or sustained diastolic pressures of 90–99 mmHg with target organ damage, evidence of established CHD, diabetes or when their ten-year CHD risk is > 15%.[84]
- A blood pressure < 140 mmHg systolic and < 85 mmHg diastolic is the recommended target after treatment for most patients.[84]

Record of practice team learning about 'coronary heart disease'
You would add the date, length of time spent, etc. on learning activity

	Activity 1: establishing and maintaining a disease register – CHD	Activity 2: reviewing practice protocols	Activity 3: targeting appropriate secondary interventions	Activity 4
In-house formal learning	Practice development manager from PCG/PCT spends 30 minutes of a practice meeting advising on new systems; followed by practice agreeing who will do what, facilitated by practice manager	Four-weekly sessions considering hypertension, angina, myocardial infarction, screening for and controlling risks of CHD: attended by GPs, nurses, practice managers. Held jointly with six neighbouring practices. Facilitated by clinical governance lead of PCG/PCT		
External courses			Practice nurse and GP attend two-day residential course on topic. Run small group session for others in practice afterwards	
Informal and personal	GPs and practice nurse read about 'how to do it' in medical weekly newspaper and discuss how suggested method would work in your practice over coffee. Later feed into in-house training (see above)	Chat together during in-house weekly sessions (see above) gives lots of food for thought. Many participants at sessions do further reading in their own time to prepare for next session		
Qualifications and/or experience gained			GP and nurse put course materials in own portfolios	

Template for your PPDP (complete one chart per topic)

What topic have you chosen?

Who chose it?

Justify why topic is a priority:

(i)   A practice and professional priority?

(ii)   A district priority?

(iii)   A national priority?

Who will be included in the practice personal and professional development plan? (give posts and names of GPs, employed staff, attached staff, others from outside the practice, patients)

Who will collect the baseline information and how?

Where are you now? (baseline)

continued overleaf

What information will you obtain about individual learning wishes and needs?
How will you obtain this and who will do it: self-completion checklists, discussion, appraisal, patient feedback?

What are the learning needs for the practice and how do they match the needs of the individual?

Patient or public input to your PPDP

How will you prioritise everyone's needs in a fair and open way? (for example, see the Hanging Committee in the example given earlier)

Aims of PPDP arising from the preliminary data-gathering exercise

---

How you might integrate the 14 components of clinical governance into your PPDP focusing on the topic of:

Establishing a learning culture:

Managing resources and services:

Establishing a research and development culture:

Reliable and accurate data:

Evidence-based practice and policy:

Confidentiality:

Health gain:

Coherent team:

Audit and evaluation:

Meaningful involvement of patients and the public:

Health promotion:

Risk management:

Accountability and performance:

Core requirements:

Action plan (include objectives, timetabled action, expected outcomes)

How does your PPDP tie in with your other strategic plans (for example the practice's business or development plan, the Primary Care Investment Plan)?

What additional resources will you require to execute your plan and from where do you hope to obtain them? (will staff have to pay any course fees or undertake learning in their own time? How much protected time will you allocate staff?)

How will you evaluate your PPDP? (who will be responsible for what?)

How will you know when you have achieved your objectives? (how will you measure success?)

How will you disseminate the learning from your plan and sustain the developments and newfound knowledge or skills?

How will you handle new learning requirements as they crop up?

Record of your learning:
Write in topic, date, time spent, type of learning

	Activity 1	Activity 2	Activity 3	Activity 4
In-house formal learning				
External courses				
Informal and personal				
Qualifications and/or experience gained				

CHAPTER EIGHT

Revalidation

How revalidation has evolved

The revalidation of doctors is well established in many countries around the world[100–102] but the concept has been slow to be introduced into the UK. The concept of a periodic, formal reassessment of a doctor's fitness to practise has long produced resentment among British GPs[103] but has now become a reality. The increasing public and media pressure that reached a head with the outcry that followed the guilty verdict passed on the mass murderer and ex-GP Harold Shipman has led to even the most recalcitrant GPs agreeing that the introduction of revalidation is inevitable and necessary.

There has been considerable activity on accreditation in general practice. There are examples of good practice throughout the UK. GP trainers have a regular review by the Directors of Postgraduate General Practice Education. These reviews allow the trainers to reflect on their practice in a supportive environment. The RCGP has been active in proposing systems of accreditation including Fellowship by Assessment, the Quality Practice Award and the team-based practice accreditation programme, all of which are voluntary.[104,105]

Work on a system of revalidation for GPs in the UK began in the early 1990s. In 1992, the General Medical Services Committee of the British Medical Association launched a consultation.[106] Over two thirds of the GPs who responded to the survey accepted the principle of revalidation. The resulting proposal of a voluntary two-level system of reaccreditation every five years was never adopted but the consultation exercise did contribute positively to the public debate.

The role of the General Medical Council

The General Medical Council (GMC) turned up the heat in 1998 when they decided unanimously that 'specialists and general practitioners must be able to demonstrate on a regular basis that they are keeping themselves up to date and remain fit to practise in their chosen field'. They set a timetable that would lead to the implementation of revalidation in 2001. They also set up a steering group to explore the practicalities of implementing their decision[107], suggesting that revalidation be linked to registration.

The public would then be assured that registered doctors had demonstrated that they remained fit to practise. The link with registration would demonstrate that the system was transparent, enabling patients to check on the status of any doctor at any time. The GMC intend the process of revalidation to be closely aligned and developed in harmony with the Government's proposals for clinical governance.[108]

The GMC has committed itself to a consultation process that is inclusive and transparent so that the final proposals will command the confidence of patients and doctors. To progress the consultation process, it established a five-tier structure beneath its Council:[109]

- revalidation steering group (only GMC members)
- external consultative group (key stakeholders)
- specialty consultative groups (doctors in training, GPs, hospital, public health)
- public and patients' consultation group
- bilateral contacts with each Royal College, government, private medicine, etc.

Details of the consultative process including reports of the meetings of the various subgroups are regularly updated on their website www.gmc-uk.org

The GMC believes that the vast majority of doctors conscientiously maintain good standards of professional practice. Revalidation should therefore be straightforward and undemanding for most doctors. It would, however, identify those doctors whose practice is in need of attention. It should also trigger a local process that would support them to improve their standards before their professional registration was put at risk. The GMC believes that the revalidation process should be a record of what a doctor is doing in practice, based on the attributes of a good doctor set out in the document *Good Medical Practice*.[110]

To this end, the GMC's revalidation steering group has constructed a framework as the basic design for the system:

- local profiling of performance
- periodic external peer review of the profiling process
- providing evidence that would lead to revalidation of the doctor's entry in the register.

These first three stages will apply to all doctors. If there is any concern about a doctor's performance then a further one or more of the following will take place:

- local remedial action
- referral to the GMC's fitness to practise procedures
- action by the GMC on the doctor's registration.

The key to the success of revalidation will be the development of the local profiling of performance. This is likely to include:

- a record of continuing educational activity
- a portfolio of wider professional development
- a record of participation in, and the results of, clinical and organisational audit

- the results of regular appraisals of the doctor's performance at work, showing any changes in the doctor's performance and set in the context of national professional standards
- an account of the views of patients and colleagues.

The plan is for the general practice profession to design a system to be put to the GMC for approval to cover the first four steps in the GMC's six-step model. The RCGP has taken a lead in bringing together the many different primary care organisations to develop proposals for all GPs.

The RCGP revalidation working group

The working group was formed in the summer of 1999 in response to the GMC's revalidation initiative. It had a wide membership that included the General Practitioners Committee of the British Medical Association (GPC); the RCGP's Patients Liaison Group and others (representatives of the RCGP, Joint Committee on Postgraduate Training for General Practice, National Association of Non-Principals, Overseas Doctors Association, Committee of General Practice Education Directors and the GMC).

The working group acknowledged that the central theme would be the GMC's publication *Good Medical Practice*.[110] A complementary document *Good Medical Practice for General Practitioners* has been produced specifically to put the GMC's guidance into the context of general practice. It was widely distributed for consultation in January 2000.[6]

The proposed content of revalidation for GPs: the evidence required

The overall standards in *Good Medical Practice for General Practitioners*:[6]

- Each GP may be asked to submit a covering statement of compliance.
- Professional relationships – maintaining trust:
  - evidence of how the GP assesses his or her communication skills and keeps them up to acceptable standards.
- Keeping up to date and maintaining performance:
  - evidence of appropriate CPD including evidence of participation in clinical audit and the PDP.
- If things go wrong:
  - evidence of an acceptable complaints procedure.
- Good clinical care:
  - evidence, for example, of the possession of appropriate diagnostic and treatment equipment.

- Keeping records and keeping colleagues informed:
  - evidence of legible and comprehensive records.
- Access and availability:
  - evidence submitted may include a copy of a patient information leaflet.
- Working with colleagues and working in teams:
  - an account of primary healthcare team communication.
- Making effective use of resources:
  - this may include submission of prescribing and activity (PACT) data.

For revalidation to be acceptable there will need to be representation from the breadth of general practice and of lay interests. While the GMC has the responsibility of determining the final structure, the proposals made by the RCGP in their consultative document chime well with the papers generated so far by the GMC (*see* Figure 8.1).

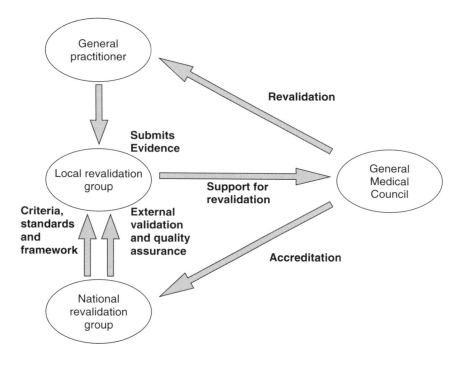

Figure 8.1   The RCGP's proposed organisation of revalidation.

When the consultation period is over, the RCGP will put forward proposals to the GMC who will make the final decision on whether their proposals are acceptable. The increasing public and governmental pressure that has built up following the Shipman verdict will undoubtedly have an effect. The Chief Medical Officer has also contributed to the debate by putting forward his own thoughts in the Department of Health's consultation document, *Supporting Doctors, Protecting Patients.*[111]

> **The principles of revalidation of professional registration are that the system must:**
>
> - be understood by and be credible with the public
> - identify unacceptable performance
> - identify good performance
> - be supported by the profession and must support the profession
> - be practical and feasible
> - not put any particular group of doctors at an advantage or a disadvantage.

Supporting Doctors, Protecting Patients

This consultation paper focused on preventing, recognising and dealing with poor clinical performance.[111] The paper acknowledged that the GMC and the Royal Colleges had made considerable progress on revalidation but expressed concern that the present NHS arrangements to investigate and deal with poor performance are seen as ineffective, slow and inadequate. It intimated that the existing arrangements did not serve the interests of patients, doctors or the NHS. The paper set out the Government's proposals to deal with the poor clinical performance of doctors in England. The paper suggested that the present management of poor performance emphasised treatment of problems rather than prevention or early intervention. Some of the proposals complemented those put forward by the GMC but some could be seen as a direct challenge to the concept of professional self-regulation and the autonomy of the GMC.

The general practice focus was on the independent contractor status and the resulting inability of health authorities to suspend GPs even in serious circumstances. The NHS Tribunal was challenged because of the perception that it is slow to reach decisions, with the result that a poorly performing doctor may continue to work and pose a danger to patients. Single-handed GPs were targeted as potential problems with their limited arrangements for peer review; but it is also acknowledged that partnerships can cover up a problem with doctors compensating for colleagues' weaknesses. It highlighted the problem with locums and other non-principals, where there is no facility to suspend them, and there is lack of support for their CPD.

The system of self-regulation at a national level must relate to clinical governance and professional responsibilities at local level for poor performance to be identified and dealt with quickly and effectively. The role of the CHI is reinforced together with the role of the NHS Executive regional offices in the performance management of the quality and standards of service delivery. The paper highlighted the existing fragmented system of self-regulation that involves a mix of mandatory and voluntary arrangements. It defined the purpose of self-regulation as being to protect the public, and set out proposals to define the basis for self-regulation by suggesting five principles of good regulation to test the appropriateness and effectiveness of regulation:

- transparency
- accountability
- targeting
- consistency
- proportionality.

The document suggested that participation in audit should be compulsory for all GPs. It proposed that education, training and CPD programmes should be reviewed to ensure that all doctors participate and that separate processes of external peer review, such as the RCGP's Fellowship by Assessment, should be encouraged and coordinated.

The report proposed that appraisal should be introduced for all doctors, with policies for addressing the needs of sick doctors and facilities for stress reduction and management training developed.

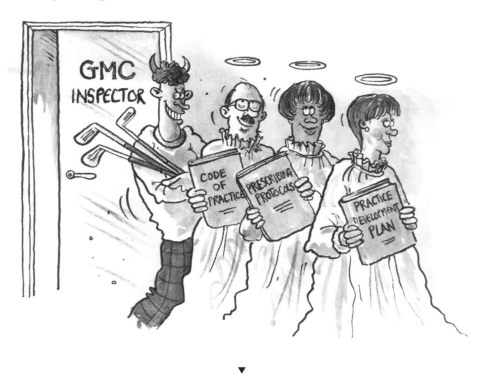

▼

The document described new mechanisms to resolve problems of poor performance, which included the development of 'Assessment and Support Centres'. They would coordinate any reskilling or retraining that a poorly performing doctor would need in close liaison with the health authority and be responsible for reassessing the doctor as fit to practise at the end of the period.

The response from general practice from the GPC, JCPTGP and RCGP[112] has been to point out that while acknowledging the problems in current management of poor performance, the arrangements proposed risk alienating the profession.

The role of PDPs and PPDPs in revalidation

One of the most important lessons to draw from the work to date on a system of revalidation is that there will be an increasing need for doctors to demonstrate their competence. This will include evidence of their participation in audit, in an appraisal system and in CPD.

The evidence will need to be collected together in a portfolio, the most important components of which will be the PPDP and the doctor's individual PDP. They will provide the evidence that the doctor has been through an appraisal process, considered his or her own learning needs, planned their learning and demonstrated the learning activity of the year before.

The responsibility for approving or accrediting the PDP will be the ultimate responsibility of the PCG/PCT's clinical governance lead but it is likely that the GP tutor will be the person actually responsible for helping the doctor produce their plan. The 'dialogue' with the GP tutor is a form of appraisal; the PDP itself is a powerful indicator of the doctor's commitment to improving the quality of their care through active participation in CPD.

CHAPTER NINE

Preparing your portfolio of evidence

Your portfolio may be useful to obtain credits for prior learning with higher degree courses at universities or to prove experience and competence in the future for revalidation of your professional qualifications, whatever your health discipline.

The steps in portfolio-based learning are:[113]

- identifying significant experiences to serve as important sources of learning
- reflecting on the learning that arose from those experiences
- demonstrating that learning in practice
- analysing the portfolio and identifying further learning needs and ways in which these needs can be met.

The portfolio may have a varied content including:

- workload logs
- audio tapes
- audit projects
- case descriptions
- patient satisfaction surveys
- a report of a change or innovation
- videos
- research surveys
- commentaries on published literature or books
- records of critical incidents and learning points
- notes from formal teaching sessions with reference to clinical work or other evidence.[114]

Analysis of the experiences and learning opportunities should show demonstrable learning outcomes and any further educational plan to meet educational needs or development still outstanding. A mentor may guide the learner as he or she compiles and analyses the material in the portfolio, providing another perspective that challenges the learner to think more deeply about their own attitudes, knowledge or beliefs. Much of the learning emanating from a portfolio is from individual reflection and self-critique in the analysis stage.[115]

There are eight steps to take to help others build up a portfolio as a GP or nurse tutor:

- develop a framework and documentation for the portfolio
- establish the means for supporting the learner during portfolio development
- introduce learners to the concept and benefits of a portfolio
- develop an individual action plan
- identify sources of evidence of learning appropriate to identified learning needs
- gather and document evidence of learning
- monitor progress. Assess/review portfolio
- use portfolio to demonstrate competence or fitness to practise.

And for someone building their own portfolio, a different perspective on those eight steps:[116]

- Write a self-appraisal action plan from the earlier information in this book. Decide where are you now? Where do you want to be in five years' time? How are you going to get there?
- Describe your approach to teaching and learning – the mix of reading and reflection, lectures, accredited courses, etc.
- Select items for inclusion for each chapter of portfolio – you might have one chapter per topic, or activity within a topic – as in the template for a PDP.
- Prepare reflective discussions for each chapter so you don't just go and sit in that lecture but pause for reflection afterwards about what you have learnt and how you'll use that learning in your everyday work, hopefully demonstrating the changes that have resulted.
- Look for gaps – in your learning, your competence, etc.
- Reflect on the original action plan – have you completed it? Have the new learning needs that have cropped up made the original plan obsolete?
- Make sure all references are complete and the evidence in your portfolio is as accurate and complete as possible.
- Share your portfolio with your mentor – could be your GP or nurse tutor, a colleague.

Evidence might be all sorts of things, not just formal audits, although they make a good start. It might include reports of educational activities attended, statements of your roles/responsibilities, copies of publications you have read or appraised, reports of your work. You could incorporate observations by others and evaluations of you observing other colleagues and how their practice differs from yours, descriptions of self-improvements, video of typical activity, materials that demonstrate your skills to others, products of your input or learning – a new protocol for example.

CHAPTER TEN

Poor performance

Setting quality standards is welcome and challenging. Enforcing them seems a difficult and perhaps threatening task. One of the main problems is how to develop quality standards and, if you do, what they will be used for. In the context of this book, the development of quality standards may be taken as:

> *A focus for individual GPs, practice nurses or groups of general practice professionals to reflect on their own practice and plan their professional development* (a definition from *Quality in General Practice*[117]).

Quality standards may also serve as:

- a framework for describing the current status of general practice at district, regional or national levels
- a means of assessing whether policy interventions (e.g. clinical governance) have been effective in raising standards
- a tool for measuring (and implicitly, penalising or rewarding) the performance of individual health professionals or practices, and recording improvement or deterioration over time
- a means of defining standards and identifying individuals, practices or health authorities who fail to meet them, i.e. a means of accountability upwards and performance management downwards
- a way of informing or justifying the allocation of limited resources to practices
- a source of information for service users.

Defining quality within a single discipline is usually done by reaching a consensus of what is 'best' practice, 'good enough' practice or 'poor' practice, and a large number of publications are referenced in *Quality in General Practice*.[117] Problems arise when different groups come together and find that each has designed their definition of quality and evaluations around different sets of underlying values and priorities.

Quality indicators that use targets need caution in their interpretation. Targets may act as disincentives (why bother at all if you think you are unlikely ever to reach them?) or be unrealistic in certain populations. They may promote inequality if efforts are directed at those who will be mostly likely to accept rather than those most in need. Targets tend to measure those things that are easy to measure, rather than patient-relevant outcomes.

NICE produces national standards based on the best evidence of the effectiveness and cost-effectiveness of different procedures. CHI will have powers to ensure that these standards are met. You need to ensure that your evidence of meeting those standards is clear, and can be demonstrated by your PCG/PCT.

Other standards will be set and, if not met, will require adequate explanation as to the reasons why not. You will need to demonstrate what action you are taking to remedy the failure as well.

One practice consistently fails to meet the lowest cervical cytology targets. After discussion with the clinical governance lead of their PCG, the practice team decides on a project to try to reach their large population of mixed ethnic minority groups, starting with contacting local opinion leaders, as part of their PPDP.

There is an upsurge of interest in developing indicators for quality in general practices and PCG/PCTs. Much work remains to be done to ensure that they are fair and representative of the views of more than one discipline. There is an expectation that comparisons within PCG/PCTs will level up standards of the 'poorest performing' general practices by peer pressure, but it remains to be seen what will happen if this does not occur.

In general practice people do not work in isolation, although some are more individualistic than others. Sooner or later episodes of poor performance will occur and require action. You need a procedure to deal with these episodes so that they can be examined and rectified, justly and honestly.

Deficiencies in the quality of performance can be listed under the three main areas:

* professional competence
* relationships with patients and colleagues
* ethical standards.

Be proactive and look at these areas critically, both for yourself and others working with you. It is best practice to use risk management to try and prevent failures before they happen.

Professional competence

Whether you work as a practice manager, receptionist, nurse, doctor, other health professional or ancillary worker, in the NHS, what you do should meet certain minimum individual professional standards. Unacceptable standards include being:

* unaware of the limits of your competence or unwilling to ask for help when those limits are reached
* a poor listener, who misses important parts of communications made to you

- unable to discuss sensitive and personal underlying matters affecting others
- unable or unwilling to explain what you are going to do or why
- poorly organised to prevent future problems, give appropriate health or safety advice, or care for long-term problems
- someone who undertakes or arranges irrelevant investigations
- someone who gives or arranges treatments that are not consistent with best practice or evidence

and being someone who fails to:

- use previous records as a source of information about past events
- examine or arrange an examination when needed
- examine or arrange an examination in an appropriate or adequate way
- have or use suitable diagnostic or treatment equipment that is in working order
- follow rational and logical thought processes from the information available, whether clinical or non-clinical
- keep up to date with current medical, nursing, legal or organisational developments
- maintain proper records and systems of review.

If you or someone you work with has any of these difficulties, look at the reasons in the same way as you would in a critical incident analysis. Decide with others if it is an important enough problem, or occurs sufficiently often, to require remedial action.

Other deficiencies that may affect the performance of the whole team or work place include the following:

- Patients have difficulty accessing medical services because of:
  - restricted opening hours, or hours that are unpredictable
  - too few unanswered or frequently engaged phone lines
  - unavailability of staff
  - poor, difficult, or unsafe access to premises or parts of premises
  - lack of information about the services available.
- Patients receive a poor quality of service because of:
  - inadequately trained staff or staff with poor levels of competence
  - lack of confidentiality
  - staff not being trained in the management of emergency situations
  - doctors or nurses not being contactable in an emergency or being ineffective
  - treatment being unavailable due to poor management of resources or services
  - poor management of the arrangements for home visiting
  - insufficient numbers of available staff for the workload
  - the qualifications of locums or deputising staff being unknown or inadequate for the post they are filling
  - the arrangements for transfer of information from one team member to another being inadequate
  - team members not acting on information received.

Many of these items will need action as a team, but for some of them, it may be your responsibility to ensure that adequate standards are met.

A patient collapsed in the waiting area after having an injection in the treatment room. The wheelchair could not be found and the hydrocortisone was found to be past its expiry date. A critical incident analysis procedure was instigated. As a result, the wheelchair was clipped to a rail by a quick release chain. The practice nurse checked the emergency drugs before each injection session and the practice manager kept a list of drugs kept in stock by the practice, and their expiry dates. She took the responsibility over from one of the doctors for reordering drugs before their expiry date. All the staff refreshed their CPR skills in a joint session run by the ambulance service. *No one person was blamed, but all staff took responsibility for the failures that had occurred and remedial action was taken.*

Relationships with patients and colleagues

In the example above, the procedure for keeping drugs up to date had been fragmented – the nurse had no procedure for regular checking. If she did notice the expiry date she would write a request on a sticky note or tell the doctor verbally. The doctor would then have to remember to tell the practice manager who would have to remember to order the drugs. The nurse, the doctor and the practice manager had each been unclear about their individual responsibilities and had just muddled through. It is important that everyone feels they can bring problems to the attention of others without fear of blame or taking or giving offence.

Colleagues and patients should be treated with respect. Good communications are essential. Procedures for reliable transmission of messages should be in place.

A patient joined a new practice. He was unable to find out from the practice leaflet what to do when he became ill at home one evening. He phoned the number on the leaflet but was unable to understand the message that gave information and then another telephone number, which was unclear. He phoned for help from his previous doctor. The new practice had the amount claimed deducted from their remuneration.

Unacceptable standards for relationships with colleagues and patients include:

*   refusing to accept patients because of prejudices against ethnic groups, the homeless, severe mental illness or other conditions
*   pressuring others to act in line with your own beliefs
*   failing to provide safeguards for the practice team when they have to see patients who pose a threat

- having no contact with, or refusing to talk to, other members of the primary care team, e.g. district nurses or health visitors
- failing to listen to the concerns of patients, relatives or staff
- being unaware of the skills of others
- delegating tasks to inappropriately or inadequately trained staff
- failing to encourage staff to develop new skills and responsibilities
- referring patients unnecessarily to others
- failing to provide sufficient information to others when referring
- paying insufficient attention to confidentiality and consent.

Some of these items require action by an individual; others require the whole team to make changes. Team meetings are often a good way of raising such concerns at an early stage.

Ethical standards

Some of the standards for professional competence and for relationships with colleagues will also have ethical implications. Poor ethical standards may also be shown by:

- giving references that are biased or untrue or omitting important information
- signing or issuing certificates or documents that contain inaccurate information without considering their implications
- not taking responsibility for your actions or performance
- ignoring other people's unacceptable performance or behaviour
- seeking personal gain over and above the normal remuneration for your work
- abusing funds provided for the care of patients
- abusing the professional trust that patients expect by inappropriate financial or personal dealings
- making poor use of the resources available (prescribing or using treatments wastefully, or not taking costs into account when managing NHS resources)
- failing to protect patients from harm in research studies or providing false data
- not taking proper responsibility for the quality of teaching when instructing others.

As you work through the identification of personal or practice learning needs, you may well come across some other items not included in the lists above. Add them to your criteria.

What should you do if you or someone else is failing to act about poor performance?

Members of teams are responsible to each other. If there is evidence of poor practice, members of the team should try to deal with it at the earliest opportunity. If you are unsure what to do, seek informal confidential advice from senior colleagues. If you *are* the senior colleague ask other colleagues whose judgement you respect.

Appraisal on a yearly basis should become normal practice for everyone who works in a general practice. The appraisal should look at individual performance over the year, including both the strengths and weaknesses. During an appraisal, the areas of poor performance should become apparent, either (preferably) identified by the person being appraised, or otherwise by the appraiser from the evidence collected. Proposals for monitoring by outside bodies make the collection of evidence, satisfactory performance or remedial action for poor performance, mandatory.

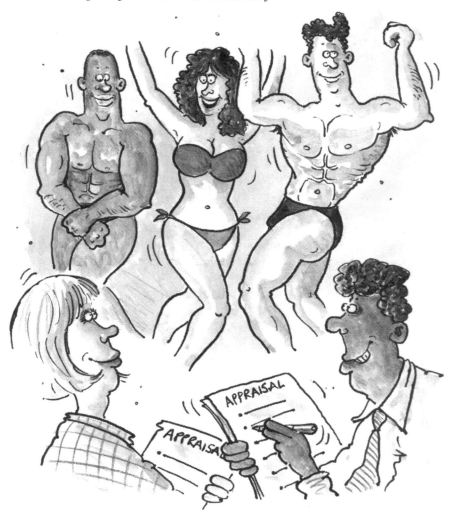

▼
Appraisal should be normal practice.

The individual or practice team may be able to sort out the problem at their own level by suitable development plans. If not, share the problem with your local medical committee, or other local colleagues who are in a position to help.

Concerns about someone's performance may come from outside the team – following complaints from patients or doubt about competence expressed by an outside professional. **Investigation to discover the facts always precedes action**.

A hospital specialist became concerned about the unusual number of diabetic patients referred to outpatients by one GP. The team investigated the comments the specialist made to the senior partner and found that the GP had become very uncertain of his management following an unexpected death. The GP agreed to make diabetes management part of his current learning plan.

Local arrangements and responsibilities will vary, but there will always be procedures that need to be followed if the problem cannot be resolved within the team framework. If there is a pattern of poor practice that, if continued, would put patients at risk, procedures should be put in place to:

- protect patients if they are at risk
- be fair
- provide support and practical help for the person or people involved.

Local action may take place within general practice with the assistance of the local medical committee, the PCG/PCT or the health authority. You should have a named local coordinator for more complex events. You may also need to consult the regional or local director of public health or the relevant professional body, e.g. the RCGP or the Royal College of Nursing. Problems with skills or knowledge may require discussion with the postgraduate dean, regional Director of Postgraduate General Practice Education or the Educational Consortia (for non-medical educational needs).

Standard local procedures are not suitable for short-term locums or professionals who may move to other parts of the country. If there are concerns about poor performance, referral to the relevant professional statutory body is necessary.

If local action fails then referral to a statutory body such as the GMC or the UKCC, etc., should be considered.

Appendix

Useful www addresses

ARIF (Aggressive Research Intelligence Facility): The University of Birmingham, 27 Highfield Road, Edgbaston, Birmingham B15 3DP. http://www.hsrc.org.uk/links/arif/arifhome.htm

Bandolier: http://www.jr2.ox.ac.uk/bandolier

CASPE (Critical Appraisal Skills Project): http://www.mailbase.ac.uk/lists/critical-appraisal-skills

CEBM (Centre for Evidence-based Medicine): http://cebm.jr2.ox.ac.uk/

The Cochrane Library. Update Software, Summertown Pavilion, Middle Way, Summertown, Oxford OX2 7LG. http://www.cochrane.co.uk or http://www.doctors.net.uk (GMC registration number required)

Healthfinder: http://www.healthfinder.org/

Medical Matrix: http://www.medmatrix.org/

Medline: http://medline.cos.com

OMNI: http://www.omni.ac.uk

STATS (Steve's Attempt To Teach Statistics): http://www.cmh.edu/stats

WISDOM (part of the Institute of General Practice and Primary Care, University of Sheffield): http://www.wisdom.org.uk

Useful publications on evidence-based practice and clinical effectiveness

Bandolier is published by the NHS Executive, Anglia and Oxford, as a monthly newsletter that describes the literature on the effectiveness of healthcare interventions in a pithy style. Moore A and McQuay H (eds), *Bandolier*, Pain Relief Unit, The Churchill, Oxford OX3 7LJ. http://www.jr2.ox.ac.uk/bandolier

Clinical Evidence. A twice-yearly compendium of the best available evidence for effective healthcare. BMJ Publishing Group. Launched in 1999.

Clinical Effectiveness Resource Pack. This resource pack is updated regularly and is produced by the NHS Executive. It includes lists of contact details for many organisations, publications and other sources of information on clinical effectiveness. There is also information about associated publications – *Effective Healthcare Bulletins, Effectiveness Matters, Epidemiologically Based Needs Assessments, Systematic Reviews of Research Evidence, Clinical Guidelines, Health Technology Assessments* and other relevant publications.

Effective Healthcare Bulletins. These bulletins are produced by the NHS Centre for Reviews and Dissemination at the University of York. They are 'based on systematic review and synthesis of research on the clinical effectiveness, cost-effectiveness and acceptability of health service interventions'.
NHS Centre for Reviews and Dissemination, University of York, York YO1 5DD. Subscriptions and copies from Royal Society of Medicine Press, PO Box 9002, London W1A 0ZA.

He@lth Information on the Internet. This is a bimonthly newsletter for all healthcare professionals published by The Royal Society of Medicine in association with the Wellcome Trust. The Royal Society of Medicine, 1 Wimpole Street, London W1M 8AE. Tel 020 7290 2927.

Health Updates from the Health Education Authority. Topics in the series are: Coronary Heart Disease, Smoking, Alcohol, Physical Activity, Workplace Health, Child Health, Immunisation. These are well-researched reference books on topical health issues. Health Education Authority, Trevelyan House, 30 Great Peter Street, London SW1P 2HW.

Woodrow P (1996) Exploring confidentiality in nursing practice. *Nursing Standard.* **10**: 38–42.

Relevant books

Baker M, Maskrey N and Kirk S (1997) *Clinical Effectiveness and Primary Care.* Radcliffe Medical Press, Oxford.
Carter Y and Thomas C (eds) (1997) *Research Methods in Primary Care.* Radcliffe Medical Press, Oxford.
Chambers R (1998) *Clinical Effectiveness Made Easy.* Radcliffe Medical Press, Oxford.
Chambers R (1999) *Involving Patients and the Public: how to do it better.* Radcliffe Medical Press, Oxford.
Chambers R, Hawksley B and Teeranlall R (1999) *Survival Skills for Nurses.* Radcliffe Medical Press, Oxford.

Chambers R and Wall D (2000) *Teaching Made Easy: a manual for health professionals.* Radcliffe Medical Press, Oxford.

Crombie I (1996) *The Pocket Guide to Critical Appraisal.* BMJ Publishing Group, London.

Deighan M and Hitch S (eds) (1995) *Clinical Effectiveness From Guidelines to Cost-effective Practice.* Earlybrave, Brentwood.

Elwyn G and Smail J (1999) *Integrated Teams in Primary Care.* Radcliffe Medical Press, Oxford.

Fry H, Ketteridge S and Marshall S (1999) *A Handbook for Teaching and Learning in Higher Education.* Kogan Page, London.

Gillies A (1999) *Information and IT for Primary Care.* Radcliffe Medical Press, Oxford.

Gray JAM (1997) *Evidence-based Healthcare.* Churchill Livingstone, Edinburgh.

Greenhalgh T (1997) *How to Read a Paper: the basics of evidence-based medicine.* BMJ Publishing Group, London.

Jones R and Menzies S (1999) *General Practice: essential facts.* Radcliffe Medical Press, Oxford.

Kiley R (1999) *Medical Information on the Internet* (2e). Harcourt Publishers Ltd, London (includes free CD-ROM).

King's Fund (1998) *Turning Evidence into Everyday Practice.* King's Fund, London.

Kobelt G (1996) *Health Economics: an introduction to economic evaluation.* Office of Health Economics, London.

Lancaster T, Straus S, Badenoch D, Richardson S *et al.* (1998) *Practising Evidence-based Medicine. Learner's Manual* (3e). Radcliffe Medical Press, Oxford.

Lilley R (1999) *Making Sense of Clinical Governance.* Radcliffe Medical Press, Oxford.

Lilley R with Davies G and Cain B (1998) *The PCG Team Builder.* Radcliffe Medical Press, Oxford.

Ling T (ed) (1999) *Reforming Healthcare by Consent.* Radcliffe Medical Press, Oxford.

Li Wan Po A (1998) *Dictionary of Evidence-based Medicine.* Radcliffe Medical Press, Oxford.

Lugon M and Secker-Walker J (1999) *Clinical Governance: making it happen.* Royal Society of Medicine Press, London.

McEvoy P (1998) *Educating the Future GP: the course organiser's handbook* (2e). Radcliffe Medical Press, Oxford.

Pike S and Forster D (1995) *Health Promotion for All.* Churchill Livingstone, Edinburgh (this book contains a framework for developing a personal health promotion portfolio).

Sackett D, Richardson S, Rosenberg W and Haynes RB (1997) *Evidence-based Medicine.* Churchill Livingstone, Edinburgh.

Strauss S, Badenoch D, Richardson S *et al.* (1998) *Practising Evidence-based Medicine. Tutor's Manual* (3e). Radcliffe Medical Press, Oxford.

Tyrrell S (1999) *Using the Internet in Healthcare.* Radcliffe Medical Press, Oxford.

van Zwanenberg T and Harrison J (eds) (2000) *Clinical Governance in Primary Care.* Radcliffe Medical Press, Oxford.

Wilson T (ed) (1999) *The PCG Development Guide.* Radcliffe Medical Press, Oxford.

References

1   Field S (2000) *Continuing Professional Development in General Practice: the regional strategy (West Midlands)*. West Midlands Postgraduate GP Education Unit, Birmingham.

2   Syder B (2000) *The Phoenix Agenda: a development framework for general practice management*. AENEAS Press, Chichester.

3   Chambers R (1999) *Involving Patients and the Public: how to do it better*. Radcliffe Medical Press, Oxford.

4   Poulton BC (1996) Use of the consultation satisfaction questionnaire to examine patients' satisfaction with general practitioners and community nurses: reliability, replicability and discriminant validity. *Br J Gen Pract.* **46**: 26–31.

5   National Primary Care Research and Development Centre (1999) General practice assessment survey. In: R Chambers *Involving Patients and the Public: how to do it better*. Radcliffe Medical Press, Oxford.

6   General Practitioners Committee and Royal College of General Practitioners (1999) *Good Medical Practice for General Practitioners*. RCGP, London.

7   Sambandan S (1999) *Surgery in the Surgery*. Radcliffe Medical Press, Oxford.

8   Greenhalgh T (1997) *How to Read a Paper*. BMJ Publishing, London.

9   Bero LA, Grilli R, Grimshaw JM *et al.* (1998) On behalf of the Cochrane Effective Practice and Organisation of Care Review Group. *BMJ.* **317**: 465–8.

10 Freemantle N, Harvey EL, Wolf F *et al.* (1999) Printed educational materials: effects on professional practice and healthcare outcomes (Cochrane Review). *The Cochrane Library*, Issue 2. Update Software, Oxford.

11 Lilley R (1999) *Making Sense of Clinical Governance*. Radcliffe Medical Press, Oxford.

12 Chambers R and Wall D (2000) *Teaching Made Easy: a manual for health professionals*. Radcliffe Medical Press, Oxford.

13 Secretary of State for Health (1998) *A First Class Service: quality in the new NHS*. Department of Health, London.

14 Department of Health (1997) *The New NHS: modern, dependable*. The Stationery Office, London.

15 Mulley A (1999) Learning from differences within the NHS. *BMJ.* **319**: 528–30.

16 Chief Nursing Officer (1998) *Integrating Theory and Practice in Nursing*. NHS Executive, London.

17 NHS Executive (1998) *Research: what's in it for consumers?* NHS Executive, Wetherby.

18 Chambers R (1998) *Clinical Effectiveness Made Easy*. Radcliffe Medical Press, Oxford.

19 Morrison J, Sullivan F, Murray E and Jolly B (1999) Evidence-based education: development of an instrument to critically appraise reports of educational interventions. *Medical Education.* **33**: 890–3.

20   Godlee F (ed) (2000) (updated every six months) *Clinical Evidence*. BMJ Publishing, London.

21   Charles R (1994) An evaluation of parent-held child health records. *Health Visitor*. **67**: 270–2.

22   Sackett DL, Rosenberg WM, Gray J *et al.* (1996) Evidence-based medicine: what it is, and what it isn't. *BMJ*. **312**: 71–2.

23   King's Fund (1997) *Turning Evidence into Everyday Practice*. King's Fund, London.

24   Carter Y and Falshaw M (eds) (1998) *Introduction to Evidence-based Primary Care and its Application in Commissioning*. An open learning programme: Evidence-based Primary Care. Radcliffe Medical Press, Oxford.

25   NHS Centre for Reviews and Dissemination (1999) Getting evidence to practice. *Effective Healthcare Bulletin*. **5**(1). Royal Society of Medicine Press, London.

26   Carter Y and Falshaw M (eds) (1998) *Finding the Papers: a guide to Medline searching*. An open learning programme: Evidence-based Primary Care. Radcliffe Medical Press, Oxford.

27   Donaldson K (ed) (1999) *Public and Professional Partnerships in Clinical Effectiveness*. Report of Conference, Scottish Clinical Resource and Audit Group (CRAG), Edinburgh.

28   Smith P (ed) (1997) *Guide to the Guidelines: disease management made simple* (3e). Radcliffe Medical Press, Oxford.

29   Miller C, Ross N and Freeman M (1999) *Shared Learning and Clinical Teamwork: new directions in education for multi-professional practice*. English National Board for Nursing, Midwifery, and Health Visiting, London.

30   Allen I (1991) *Family Planning and Pregnancy Counselling for Young People*. Policy Studies Institute, London.

31   Glen S (1997) Confidentiality: a critique of the traditional view. *Nursing Ethics*. **4**: 403–6.

32   Department of Health (1997) *Report of the Review of Patient-identifiable Information*. In: The Caldicott Committee Report. Department of Health, London.

33   Jacobson B, Smith A and Whitehead M (1991) *The Nation's Health: a strategy for the 1990s*. King Edward's Hospital Fund for London, London.

34   Black D (chair) (1980) *Inequalities in Health*. Report of a research working group. DHSS, London.

35   Whitehead M (1988) The health divide. In: *Inequalities in Health*. Penguin, London.

36   Nardone A, Mercey DE and Johnson AM (1997) Surveillance of sexual behaviour among homosexual men in a Central London Health Authority. *Genitourinary Medicine*. **73**: 198–202.

37   Lancaster T, Silagy C, Fowler G and Spiers I (1999) Training health professionals in smoking cessation. In: *The Cochrane Library*. Update Software, Oxford.

38   Wilson JMG (1976) Some principles of early diagnosis and detection. In: G Teeling-Smith (ed) *Proceedings of a Colloquium: Magdalen College, Oxford*. Office of Health Economics, London.

39   Clarke R and Croft P (1998) *Critical Reading for the Reflective Practitioner*. Butterworth-Heinemann, Oxford.

40   Dunning M *et al.* (1999) *Experience, Evidence and Everyday Practice*. King's Fund, London.

41 Coffey T, Boersma G, Smith L and Wallace P (eds) (1999) *Visions of Primary Care*. King's Fund, London.

42 NHS Executive (1999) *Clinical Governance: quality in the new NHS*. NHS Executive, London.

43 Poulton B and West M (1999) The determinants of effectiveness in primary healthcare teams. *J Interprof Care*. **13**(1): 7–18.

44 Chambers R and Davies M (1999) *What Stress in Primary Care!* Royal College of General Practitioners, London.

45 Elwyn G and Smail J (1998) *Integrated Teams in Primary Care*. Radcliffe Medical Press, Oxford.

46 Irvine D and Irvine S (eds) (1997) *Making Sense of Audit* (2e). Radcliffe Medical Press, Oxford. (Out of print.)

47 Donabedian A (1966) Evaluating the quality of medical care. *Millbank Memorial Fund Quarterly*. **44**: 166–204.

48 NHS Executive (1996) *Clinical Audit in the NHS. Using clinical audit in the NHS: a position statement*. NHS Executive, Leeds.

49 Maxwell R (1984) Quality assessment in health. *BMJ*. **288**: 1470–2.

50 Firth-Cozens J (1993) *Audit in Mental Health Services*. LEA, Hove.

51 NHS Executive (1997) *Priorities and Planning Guidelines for the NHS; medium-term priorities*. The Stationery Office, London.

52 Naidoo J and Wills J (1994) *Health Promotion: foundations for practice*. Baillière Tindall, London.

53 Beattie A (1991) In: J Gabe, M Calnan and M Bury (eds) *The Sociology of the Health Service*. Routledge, London.

54 Higson N (1996) *Risk Management: health and safety in primary care*. Butterworth-Heinemann, Oxford.

55 Pligt J (1998) Perceived risk and vulnerability as predictors of precautionary behaviour. *Br J Health Psychology*. **3**: 1–14.

56 Carter Y and Thomas C (1997) *Research Methods in Primary Care*. Radcliffe Medical Press, Oxford.

57 Grant J, Chambers E and Jackson G (1999) *The Good CPD Guide*. Read Healthcare, Sutton.

58 Scrivens E (1998) Policy issues in accreditation. *Int J Quality Healthcare*. **10**(1): 1–5.

59 NHS Executive (1999) *The NHS Performance Assessment Framework*. DoH, London.

60 NHS Executive (1999) *Quality and Performance in the NHS: clinical indicators*. NHS Executive, Leeds.

61 Roland M (1999) Quality and efficiency: enemies or partners? *Br J Gen Pract*. **49**: 140–3.

62 Rajaratnum G (1999) *Prioritising Health and Healthcare in North Staffordshire: a proposal to establish a North Staffordshire Priorities Forum*. North Staffordshire Health Authority, Stoke-on-Trent.

63 Calpin-Davies PJ and Akehurst RL (1999) Doctor–nurse substitution: the workforce equation. *J Nurse Management*. **7**: 71–9.

64 Wilson T, Butler F and Watson M (1998) Establishing educational needs in a new organisation. *Career Focus/BMJ.* **317**: 2–3.

65 Chambers R and Schrijver E (2000) Making practice-based professional development plans relevant to service needs and priorities. *Education for General Practice* (in press).

66 Moloney R, Macleod N and Chambers R (1999) *The Education and Training Needs of PCGs.* Staffordshire University, Stoke-on-Trent.

67 Feather A and Fry H (1999) Key aspects of teaching and learning in medicine and dentistry. In: H Fry, S Ketteridge and S Marshall (eds) *A Handbook for Teaching and Learning in Higher Education.* Kogan Page, London.

68 Roland M, Holden J and Campbell S (1999) *Quality Assessment for General Practice: supporting clinical governance in PCGs.* National Primary Care Research and Development Centre, University of Manchester, Manchester.

69 Standing Committee on Postgraduate Medical and Dental Education (1997) *Multi-professional Working and Learning: sharing the educational challenge.* SCOPME, London.

70 Miller C, Ross N and Freeman M (1999) *Researching Professional Education.* Research reports series No. 14. English National Board for Nursing, Midwifery and Health Visiting, Cambridge.

71 Audit Commission (2000) *Forget Me Not.* Audit Commission, London.

72 Drugs and Therapeutics Bulletin (2000) Rivastigmine for Alzheimer's disease. *Drugs and Therapeutics Bulletin.* **38**(2): 15–16.

73 Doyle F (1999) *Dementia.* The RCGP Members' Reference Book 1999/2000. Campden Publishing, London.

74 Corrada M, Brookmeyer R and Kawas C (1995) Sources of variability in prevalence rates of Alzheimer's Disease. *Int J of Epidemiology* **24**(5): 1000–5.

75 Folstein MF, Folstein SE and McHugh PR (1975) 'Mini-Mental State'. A practical method for grading the cognitive state of patients for the clinicians. *J Psychiatr Res.* **12**: 189–98.

76 Walstar GJ (1997) Reversible dementia in elderly patients referred to a memory clinic. *J Neurol.* **244**(1): 17–22.

77 Kiley R (1999) *Medical Information on the Internet* (2e). Churchill Livingstone, London.

78 The Informatics Review on-line lessons in Clinical Informatics http://www.informatics-review.com/lessons.html

79 Grant RM, Horkin EJ, Melhuish PJ *et al.* (1998) Different approaches to the tasks of educating and training information system professionals, within the National Health Service (UK). *Int J Med Inf.* **50**: 171–7.

80 NHS192 is found at http://www.nhspeople.net or via fax on 0114 235 1345 or email info@nhspeople.net

81 Department of Health (1999) *Mental Health. National Service Framework.* Department of Health, London.

82 Department of Health (1999) *Saving Lives. Our Healthier Nation.* The Stationery Office, London.

83 Smith P (ed) (1997) *Guide to the Guidelines* (3e). Radcliffe Medical Press, Oxford.

84   Foord-Kelcey G (ed) (2000) *Guidelines: summarising clinical guidelines for primary care.* Medendium Publishing Group, Herts.

85   Godlee F (ed) (1999) *Clinical Evidence.* Issue 2. BMJ Publishing Group, London.

86   Department of Health (1999) *Back in Work Information Document.* Health Education Authority, London.

87   McCormick A, Fleming D, Charlton J (1995) *Morbidity Statistics from General Practice. Fourth national study 1991–92.* Office of Population Censuses and Surveys, London.

88   Clinical Standards Advisory Group (1994) *Epidemiology Review: the epidemiology and cost of back pain.* The Stationery Office, London.

89   Department of Health Statistics Division (1999) *The Prevalence of Back Pain in Great Britain in 1998.* Office of National Statistics, The Stationery Office, London.

90   Thomas E, Silman A, Croft P *et al.* (1999) Predicting who develops chronic low back pain in primary care: a prospective study. *BMJ.* **318**: 1662–7.

91   Waddell G, McIntosh A, Hutchinson A *et al.* (1999) *Low back pain evidence review.* Royal College of General Practitioners, London.

92   Social Exclusion Unit (1999) *Teenage Pregnancy.* The Stationery Office, London.

93   Effective Healthcare Bulletin (1997) *Preventing and Reducing the Adverse Effects of Unintended Teenage Pregnancies.* NHS Centre for Reviews and Dissemination, University of York.

94   Meyrick J and Swann C (1998) *An Overview of the Effectiveness of Interventions and Programmes Aimed at Reducing Unintended Conceptions in Young People.* Health Education Authority, London.

95   Acheson D (1998) *Independent Inquiry into Inequalities in Health.* The Stationery Office, London.

96   Clinical Evidence Team and Advisers (1999) *Clinical Evidence.* BMJ Publishing Group, London.

97   Herman WH (1999) Glycaemic control in diabetes. *BMJ.* **319**: 104–6.

98   Whelton PK, Appel LJ, Espeland MA *et al.* (1998) Sodium reduction and weight loss in the treatment of hypertension of older persons. *JAMA.* **279**: 839–46.

99   Wood M (1999) SMAC guidelines pave the way for effective use of statins. *Guidelines in Practice.* **2**: 41–6.

100   Hays RB, Bridges-Webb C and Booth B (1993) Quality assurance in general practice. *Medical Education.* **27**: 175–80.

101   Gellhorn A (1991) Periodic physician recredentialling. *JAMA.* **265**: 752–5.

102   McAuley RG and Henderson HW (1984) Results of the peer assessment program of the College of Physicians and Surgeons of Ontario. *Can Med Assoc J.* **131**: 557–61.

103   Nicol F (1995) Making reaccreditation meaningful (discussion paper). *Br J Gen Pract.* **45**: 321–4.

104   Birch K, Field SJ and Scrivens E (2000) *Quality in General Practice.* Radcliffe Medical Press, Oxford.

105   Walsh N and Walshe K (1998) *Accreditation in Primary Care*. University of Birmingham, Birmingham.

106   General Medical Services Committee (1992) *Your Choices for the Future*. General Medical Services Committee, London.

107   General Medical Council (1999) *Revalidation: the profession moves forward*. General Medical Council News Issue 5. General Medical Council, London.

108   General Medical Council (1999) *Report of the Revalidation Steering Group, February 1999*. General Medical Council, London.

109   General Medical Council (1999) *Progress Report on the Development of Revalidation Proposals, November 1999*. General Medical Council, London.

110   General Medical Council (1995) *Good Medical Practice*. General Medical Council, London.

111   Department of Health (1999) *Supporting Doctors, Protecting Patients*. Department of Health, London.

112   Royal College of General Practitioners (2000) *Response to 'Supporting Doctors, Protecting Patients'*. Royal College of General Practitioners, London.

113   Royal College of General Practitioners (1993) *Portfolio-based Learning in General Practice*. Occasional Paper 63. RCGP, London.

114   Woodrow M (1999) The struggle for the soul of lifelong learning. *Widening Participation and Lifelong Learning*. **1**(1): 9–12.

115   Challis M (1999) AMEE Medical education guide No. 11 (revised): portfolio-based learning and assessment in medical education. *Medical Teacher*. **21**(4): 370–86.

116   Mathers N, Challis M, Howe A *et al.* (1999) Portfolios in continuing medical education – effective and efficient? *Medical Education*. **33**: 521–30.

117   Greenhalgh T and Eversley J (1999) *Quality in General Practice*. King's Fund, London.

Index